Evaluation and Management

Coding Made Easy

2024

Terry Tropin, MSHAI, RHIA, CCS-P

AHIMA-Approved ICD-10-CM/PCS Trainer

To my family – Zee, Doodle and Jazzy, for their support and love

Reviewers

Aylin Edelman, MD, RHIA, CCS

Lois Freedman, RHIT, CCS

Suzanne Lasky, CPC

Miroslava Rudneva, MS, RHIT, CCS, COBGC

Filipe Telles, RHIT, CCS

Table of Contents

Introduction

Many people find Evaluation and Management (E/M) services the most confusing part of Current Procedural Terminology (CPT®) coding, particularly with the extensive changes made to the guidelines over the last few years. Important guidelines are buried in long introductions to sections, and many terms are either strictly defined or not defined at all. Many codes are not in numerical order. Determining the levels of service is particularly confusing.

This book combines all guidelines related to an E/M service together into charts for easy reference.

Chapter 1 discusses the components used to determine most codes: an appropriate history and examination (as determined by the provider); medical decision making (MDM); time spent with the patient; age of the patient; or other criteria. Many codes use multiple criteria.

Chapters 2-15 discuss each category of codes (outpatient, inpatient, emergency department, etc.) in detail, including those that are selected using medical decision making and time, and those that are not.

These chapters describe specific categories of codes, including a summary of the codes in this category, specific levels of medical decision making and time for each code in the category, and guidelines for using these codes.

The chapters summarize the code category and includes these headings:
- General Guidelines
- Patients
- Providers
- Selecting codes using time and/or MDM
- Encounters (initial, subsequent, discharge services)
- Multiple Settings
- Multiple Providers
- Other Services (services included and not included in the category of codes)

Not all code categories will include all these headings.

Chapter 18 describes modifiers used with E/M codes.

Chapter 19 defines terms used in E/M codes.

At the end of each chapter are quizzes to check your understanding. The answers to the quizzes are in Appendix B.

Appendix A includes a form that can be used to help select the appropriate code.

This publication is designed for use as a supplement to coding textbooks for students and as a quick reference for coders already working in the field. It is **NOT** designed as a complete textbook on CPT coding. Coders should confirm the code selected using the CPT code book.

Following is a summary of the codes and the factors are used to select the correct code.

Summary of E/M Codes

Codes		Correct Code Determined by -			
		Medically appropriate history and/or examination	MDM	Time	Other Criteria
99202-99205, 99211-99215	Office/other outpatient services	√	√	√	New or Established patients
99221-99223, 99231-99233	Hospital inpatient or observation care	√	√	√	Initial or Subsequent encounter
99234-99236	Hospital inpatient or observation care services (Including admission and discharge services)	√	√	√	
99238, 99239	Hospital discharge management			√	
99242-99245, 99252-99255	Consultations	√	√	√	Inpatient/observation or outpatient
99281-99285	Emergency department services	√	√		
99288	Direction of emergency medical system (EMS) care, advanced life support				Specific services listed in introduction to this section
99291, +99292	Critical care services			√	
99304-99310	Nursing facility services	√	√	√	Initial or Subsequent encounter
99315-99316	Nursing facility discharge services			√	
99341, 99442, 99344, 99345, 99347-99350	Home or residence services	√	√	√	New or Established patient
99358, +99359	Prolonged services on date other than face-to-face service			√	Indirect patient contact (non-face-to-face services)
99360	Standby services			√	
99366-99368	Medical team conferences			√	Age of patient Direct or Indirect patient contact (face-to-face or non-face-to-face)
99374-99380	Care plan oversight services			√	Location of patient

(continued on next page)

Summary of E/M Codes (continued)

Codes		Correct Code Determined by -			
		Medically appropriate history and/or examination	MDM	Time	Other Criteria
99381-99387, 99391-99397	Preventive medicine				Age of patient New or Established patient
99401-99404, 99406-99409, 99411, 99412	Counseling and risk factor reduction and behavioral change intervention			√	Group or Individual counseling
+99415, +99416	Prolonged clinical staff services			√	Direct patient contact (face-to-face services)
+99417, +99418	Prolonged outpatient services on same date as other E/M service			√	Indirect patient contact (non-face-to-face services)
99421-99423	Online digital E/M services			√	Established patient only
99424-99427	Principal care management services			√	
99441-99443	Telephone services			√	Indirect patient contact (non-face-to-face services)
99446-99452	Interprofessional telephone/internet/ electronic health record consultations			√	Provider either consultant or treating/ requesting provider
99453, 99454, 99091, 99473-99474	Digitally stored data service/remote physiologic monitoring			√	Specific services listed in codes
99457, +99458	Remote physiologic monitoring treatment management services			√	
99450	Basic life and/or dis-ability evaluation services				Specific services listed in codes
99455, 99456	Work related/medical disability evaluation services				Specific services listed in codes
99460-99463	Newborn care services				Location of patient Initial or Subsequent encounter
99464, 99465	Delivery/birthing room attendance and resuscitation services				Specific services listed in codes

(continued on next page)

9

Summary of E/M Codes (continued)

Codes		Correct Code Determined by -			
		Medically appropriate history and/or examination	MDM	Time	Other Criteria
99466-99472, 99485, +99486	Pediatric critical care patient transport			√	Age of patient, Face-to-face or via 2-way communication
99468, 99469, 99471, 99472, 99475, 99476	Inpatient neonatal and pediatric critical care				Initial or subsequent encounter
99477-99480	Intensive neonatal care				Age of patient, Initial or Subsequent encounter
99483	Cognitive assessment and care plan services				Specific services listed in code
99484	General behavioral health integration care management				Specific services listed in codes
99487, +99489	Complex chronic care management services			√	Specific services listed in code
99490, 99491, +99437, +99439	Chronic care management services			√	Specific services listed in code
99492, 99493, +99494	Psychiatric collaborative care management services			√	Specific services listed in codes
99495, 99496	Transitional care management services		√		Specific services listed in codes
99497, +99498	Advance care planning			√	Specific services listed in codes

Summary of Changes to CPT® Evaluation and Management Codes 2024

Following is a summary of the changes to Evaluation and Management Services for 2024. New wording is <u>underlined</u>; deleted wording is ~~crossed out~~.

The most important change concerns the times listed within the codes.

Changes were made to the times listed for the office or other outpatient codes. Previously, the times were listed as ranges. For 2024, the times are listed a specific number of minutes. This makes this section consistent with other E/M categories. The wording for the codes was also revised. For example:

> **99204** Office or other outpatient visit for the evaluation and management of a new patient, which requires a medically appropriate history and/or examination and moderate level of medical decision making.
>
> When using <u>total</u> time on the date <u>of the encounter</u> for code selection, 45 ~~59 minutes of total time is spent on the date of the encounter~~ minutes must be met or exceeded.

Times were also changed for some nursing facility codes:

> **99306** Initial nursing facility care, per day, for the evaluation and management of a patient, which requires a medically appropriate history and/or examination and high level of medical decision making.
>
> When using total time on the date of the encounter for code selection, ~~45~~ 50 minutes must be met or exceeded.
>
> **99308** Subsequent nursing facility care per day for the evaluation and management of a patient, which requires a medically appropriate history and/or examination and low level of medical decision making.
>
> When using total time on the date of the encounter for code selection, ~~15~~ 20 minutes must be met or exceeded.

Changes were also made to these sections:
- Introduction - Instructions for use of the CPT codebook
- Evaluation and Management Services Guidelines
- Specific categories of E/M services
- New Code

<u>Instructions for Use of the CPT Codebook.</u>

1. New section - <u>Audio-video (Appendix P) and Audio-Only (Appendix T) Telemedicine Services Criteria</u>

   <u>The following criteria are used by the Current Procedural Terminology/Health Care Professional Advisor Committee (CPT/HCPAC) and the CPT Editorial Panel for evaluating inclusion of services in Appendix P (synchronous audio-video) and Appendix T (synchronous audio-only) telemedicine services. Any request for inclusion in Appendix P and Appendix T must satisfy the following criteria:</u>

- The totality and quality of the communication of information exchanged between the physician or other qualified healthcare provide (QHP) and the patient during the synchronous telemedicine service must be of an amount and a nature that would be sufficient to meet the requirements for the same service if services were to be rendered during an in-person face-to-face interaction; *And*
- The evidence supports the benefits of performing the service through telecommunications technology. These benefits may include, but are not limited to, the following;
  - Facilitate a diagnosis or treatment plan that may reduce complications
  - Decrease diagnostic or therapeutic interventions
  - Decrease hospitalizations
  - Decrease in-person visits to physician or other QHP office, including urgent care centers
  - Increase rapidity of resolution
  - Decrease quantifiable symptoms
  - Reduce recovery time
  - Enhance access to care, such as for rural and vulnerable patients; *and*
- A service is ineligible for inclusion in Appendix T without also being requested for inclusion, or has current inclusion, in Appendix P.

  (For a listing of CPT codes that may be used for synchronous real-time interactive audio-video telemedicine services when appended with modifier 95, see Appendix P)
  (For a listing of CPT codes that may be used for synchronous real-time interactive audio-only telemedicine services when appended with modifier 93, see Appendix T).

2. Revisions were made to the section entitled: Time
   The CPT code set contains many codes with a time basis for code selection. The following standards shall apply to time measurement, unless there are code or code-range-specific instructions in guidelines, parenthetical instructions, or code descriptions to the contrary. Time is the face-to-face time with the patient…. A unit of time is attained when the mid-point is passed. For example, an hour is attained when 31 minutes have elapsed (more than midway between zero and 60 minutes). A second hour is attained when a total of 91 minutes has elapsed. ~~When codes are ranked in sequential typical time and the actual time is between two typical times, the code with the actual time is between two typical times, the code with the typical time closest to the actual time is used. See also~~ The evaluation and management codes (E/M) codes that use total time on the date of the encounter have a required time threshold for time-based reporting; therefore, the mid-point concept does not apply. See also the Evaluation and Management (E/M) Services Guidelines…

General Evaluation and Management Services Guidelines

Changes were made to guidelines related to split or shared visits, multiple E/M services on the same date and selecting a level of service based on time. In addition, one new code was added.

1. The section on **Split or Shared Visits** was moved and revised. The section was previously included in paragraph under heading Guidelines for Selecting Level of Services Based on Time. For 2024, it is now a separate section.
   ~~A shared or split visit is defined as a visit in which a~~ Physician(s) and other qualified healthcare professional(s) ~~both provide the face-to-face and non-face-to-face work related to the visit~~ working together during a single E/M service.
   The split or shared visits guidelines are applied to determine which professional may report the service. If the physician or other QHP performs a substantive portion of the encounter, the physician or other QHP may report the service.

If code selection is based on total time on the date of the encounter, the service is reported by the professional who spent the majority of the face-to-face or non-face-to-face time performing the service.

~~When time is being used to select the appropriate level of services for which time-based reporting or shared or split visits is allowed, the time personally spent by the physician and other qualified health care professionals) assessing and managing the patient and/or counseling, educating, communicating results to the patient/family/caregiver on the date of the encounter is summed to define total time.~~

~~Only distinct time should be summed for shared or split visits (ie, when two or more individuals jointly meet with or discuss the patient, only the time of one individual should be counted.)~~

For the purpose of reporting E/M services within the context of team-based care, performance of a substantive part of the MDM requires that the physician(s) or other QHP(s) made or approved the management plan for the **_number and complexity of problems addressed at the encounter_** and takes responsibility for that plan with its inherent **_risk of complications and/or morbidity or mortality of patient management_**. By doing so, a physician or other QHP has performed two of the three elements used in the selection of the code level based on MDM.

If **_the amount and/or complexity of data to be reviewed and analyzed_** is used by the physician or other QHP to determine the reported code level, assessing an independent historian's narrative and the ordering or review of tests or documents do not have to be personally performed by the physician or other QHP, because the relevant items would be considered in formulating the management plan. Independent interpretation of tests and discussion of management plan or test interpretation must be personally performed by the physician or other QHP if these are used to determine the reported code level by the physician or other QHP.

2. A new section was also added related to **Multiple Evaluation and Management Services on the Same Date**

    The following guidelines apply to services that a patient may receive for hospital inpatient care, observation care, or nursing facility care. For instructions regarding transitions to these settings from the office or outpatient, home or residence, or emergency department setting, see guidelines for **Hospital Inpatient and Observation Care Services** or **Nursing Facility Services**.

    A patient may receive E/M services in more than one setting on a calendar date. A patient may also have more than one visit in the same setting on a calendar date. The guidelines for multiple E/M services on the same date address circumstances in which the patient has received multiple visits or services from the same physician or other QHP or another physician or other QHP of the exact same specialty and subspecialty who belongs to the same group practice.

    Per day: The hospital inpatient and observation care services and the nursing facility services are "per day" services. When multiple visits occur over the course of a single calendar date in the same setting, a single service is reported. When using MDM for code level selection, use the aggregated MDM over the course of the calendar date. When using time for code level selection, sum the time over the course of the day using the guidelines for reporting time.

13

Multiple encounters in different settings or facilities: A patient may be seen and treated in different facilities (eg, a hospital-to-hospital transfer).
When more than one primary E/M service is reported and time is used to select the code level for either service, only the time spent providing that individual service may be allocated to the code level selected for reporting that service. No time may be counted twice when reporting more than one E/M service.

Prolonged services are also based on the same allocation and their relationship to the primary service. The designation of the facility may be defined by licensure or regulation. Transfer from a hospital bed to a nursing facility bed in a hospital with nursing facility beds is considered as two services in two facilities because there is a discharge from one type of designation to another. An intra-facility transfer for a different level of care (eg, from a routine unit to a critical care unit) does not constitute a new stay, nor does it constitute a transfer to a different facility.

Emergency department (ED) and services in other settings (same or different facilities): Time spent in an ED by a physician or other QHP who provides subsequent E/M services may be included in calculating total time on the date of the encounter when ED services are not reported and another E/M service is reported (eg, hospital inpatient and observation care services).

Discharge services and services in other facilities: Each service may be reported separately as long as any time spent on the discharge service is not counted towards the total time of a subsequent service in which code level selection for the subsequent service is based on time. This includes any hospital inpatient or observation care services (including admission and discharge services) time (99234, 99235, 99236) because these services may be selected based on MDM or time.

When these services are reported with another E/M service on the same calendar date, time related to the hospital inpatient or observation care service (including admission and discharge services) may not be used for code selection of the subsequent service.

Discharge services and services in the same facility: If the patient is discharged and readmitted to the same facility on the same calendar date, report a subsequent care service instead of a discharge or initial service. For the purpose of E/M reporting, this is a single stay.

Discharge services and services in a different facility: If the patient is admitted to another facility, for the purpose of E/M reporting this is considered a different stay. Discharge and initial services may be reported as long as time spent on the discharge service is not counted towards the total time of the subsequent service reported when code level selection is based on time.

Critical care services (including neonatal intensive care services and pediatric and neonatal critical care): Reporting guidelines for intensive and critical care services that are performed on the same calendar date as another E/M service are described in the service specific section guidelines.

Transitions between office or other outpatient, home or residence, or emergency department and hospital inpatient or observation or nursing facility: See the guidelines for **Hospital Inpatient and Observation Care Services** or **Nursing Facility Services**. If the patient is seen in two settings and only one service is reported, the total time on the date of the encounter or the aggregated MDM is used for determining the level of the single reported service. If prolonged services are reported, use the prolonged services code that is appropriate for the primary service reported, regardless of where the patient was located when the prolonged services time threshold was met. The choice of the primary service is at the discretion of the reporting physician or other QHP.

3. Section revised: Guidelines for Selecting Level of Service Based on Time

   Paragraphs added: Each service that may be reported using time for code level selection has a required time threshold. The concept of attaining a mid-point between levels does not apply. A full 15 minutes is required to report any unit of prolonged services codes 99417, 99418.

   Physician(s) and other qualified health care professional(s) may each provide a portion of the face-to-face and non-face-to-face work related to the service. When time is being used to select the appropriate level of services for which time-based reporting is allowed, the time personally spent by the physician(s) and other qualified health care professional(s) assessing and managing the patient and/or counseling, educating, communicating results to the patient/family/caregiver on the date of the encounter is summed to define total time. Only distinct time should be summed (ie, when two or more individuals jointly meet with or discuss the patient, only the time of one individual should be counted).

Guidelines for Specific Sections of E/M Codes

Changes were made to these sections: initial hospital inpatient or observation care and prolonged services codes.

1. Initial hospital inpatient or observation care

   The guidelines for the section initial Hospital Inpatient or Observation Care were revised: If a consultation is performed in anticipation of, or related to, an admission by another physician or other qualified health care professional, and then the same consultant performs an encounter once the patient is admitted by the other physician or other qualified health care professional, report the consultant's inpatient encounter with the appropriate subsequent care code….This instruction applies whether the consultation occurred on the date of the admission or a date previous to the admission. It also applies…

   Changes were also made to the guidelines for codes for same day admission and discharge services.

   Added to paragraph 1: The following codes are used to report hospital inpatient or observation care services provided to patents admitted and discharged on the same date or service when the stay is more than eight hours. These services are only used by the physician or other qualified health care professional team who performs both the initial and discharge services. Other physicians and other qualified health care professionals may report 99221, 99222, 99223, as appropriate.

   When a patient receives hospital inpatient or observation care for fewer than eight hours, only the initial hospital inpatient or observation care codes…may be reported for the date of admission. Hospital or observation discharge day management codes …may not be reported. When a patient receives hospital inpatient or observation care for a minimum of eight hours and is discharged on the same calendar date, observation or inpatient care services (including admission and discharge services) codes…may be reported. Codes 99238, 99239 are not reported.

   New table added for reporting these codes based on length of stay on same date Added note under code 99239: (Do not report 99238, 99239 in conjunction with 99221, 99222, 99223 for admission and discharge services performed on the same date.)

2. Prolonged Services With or Without Direct Patient Contact on the Date of an Evaluation and Management Service

Added to first paragraph: Cognitive assessment and care plan services code 99483 does not have a required time threshold, and 99417 may be reported when the typical time has been exceeded by 15 minutes.

New note under 99417:
(Use 99417 in conjunction with 99483, when the total time on the date of the encounter exceeds the typical time of 99483 by 15 minutes or more)
Tables added and revised for coding listed with prolonged services with or without direct patient contact on the date of an E/M service and reorganized - added 99233, 99233, 99255, 99306, 99310, 99345, 99350, 99483

3. Digitally Stored Data Services/Remote Physiologic Monitoring

Note added under 99453 – (Do not report 99453 in conjunction with 0811T)

Note added under 99454 – (Do not report 99454 in conjunction with 0812T)

New Codes

A new code was added: 99459 Pelvic examination (List separately in addition to code for primary procedure)

A new add-on code was added for Medicare patients (but may be utilized by other payers): G2211 Office and Outpatient E/M visit complexity. This code can be used with codes 99202-99205, 99211-99215, regardless of the provider's specialty.

Chapter 1

Selecting a CPT® Evaluation and Management Code

Most Evaluation and Management (E/M) codes are selected by medical decision making (MDM) or time spent with the patient. This chapter discusses each of these components in detail.

Summary of Criteria Used to Select Evaluation and Management Codes

Codes		Correct Code Determined by -		
		Medically appropriate history and/or examination	MDM	Time
99202-99205, 99211-99215	Office/other outpatient services	√	√	√
99221-99223, 99231, 99233	Hospital inpatient or observation care	√	√	√
99234-99236	Hospital inpatient or observation care services (Including admission and discharge services)	√	√	√
99238, 99239	Hospital discharge management			√
99242-99245, 99252-99255	Consultations	√	√	√
99281-99285	Emergency department services	√	√	
99291, +99292	Critical care services			√
99304-99310	Nursing facility services	√	√	√
99315, 99316	Nursing facility discharge management			√
99341-99345, 99347-99350	Home or residence services	√	√	√
99358. +99359	Prolonged services			√
99360	Standby services			√
99366-99368	Medical team conferences			√
99374-99380	Care plan oversight services			√
99401-99404, 99406-99409, 99411, 99412	Counseling and risk factor reduction and behavioral change intervention			√

(continued on next page)

Summary of Criteria Used to Select Evaluation and Management Codes (continued)

Codes		Correct Code Determined by -		
		Medically appropriate history and/or examination	MDM	Time
+99415, +99416	Prolonged clinical staff services			√
+99417, +99418	Prolonged outpatient services on same date as other E/M service			√
99421-99423	Online digital services			√
99424-99427	Principal care management services			√
99441-99443	Telephone services			√
99446-99452	Interprofessional telephone/internet/ electronic health record consultations			√
99453, 99454, 99091, 99473, 99474	Digitally stored data service/remote physiologic monitoring			√
99457, 99458	Remote physiologic monitoring treatment management services			√
99466, +99467, 99485, +99486	Pediatric critical care patient transport			√
99487-+99489	Complex chronic care management services			√
99490, 99491, +99437, +99439	Chronic care management services			√
99492, 99493, +99494	Psychiatric collaborative care management services			√
99495, 99496	Transitional care management services		√	
99497, +99498	Advance care planning			√

Each category or subcategory of E/M service (eg, office or outpatient, emergency department) includes from three to five different levels in different categories of codes. Levels are **NOT** Interchangeable among the different categories or subcategories.

For example, the first level of E/M services in the subcategory of office visit, <u>new patient</u>, does **NOT** have the same requirements for medical decision making and time as the first level of E/M services in the subcategory of office visit, <u>established patient</u>.

See Appendix A for a form to assist in selecting an E/M code using these factors.

Codes may also be selected according to:
- Patient status (new or established) or
- Timing of encounter (initial or subsequent), or
- Location of encounter (outpatient, consultation, nursing facility).

For definitions of types of providers, new/established patients, initial/subsequent services, and other terms used in CPT code book and in this book, see chapter 19.

Medically Appropriate History and/or Examination

Many codes state that a medically appropriate history and/or examination, when performed, are included in the service. What is considered an appropriate history and examination is not defined.

The treating physician or other qualified health care professional who is reporting the service determines what is an appropriate history and/or examination for a specific patient. These are **NOT** elements used in selection of the level of an E/M services code even when mentioned in a code description.

The care team may collect information, and the patient or caregiver may supply information directly (eg, by electronic health record [EHR] portal or questionnaire) that is reviewed by the reporting physician or other qualified health care professional.

In most cases, code selection is based on time or medical decision making (MDM), not history and examination. Time and MDM are discussed on the following pages.

For codes selected using either time or medical decision making, use the code for the higher level of service.

For example, a subsequent hospital observation service is documented as 25 minutes with moderate medical decision making. The time is represented by code 99231 (25 minutes, straightforward or low MDM), but the MDM is represented by code 99232 (35 minutes, moderate MDM). Report code 99232 which represents the higher level of service and will be reimbursed at a higher amount.

Medical Decision Making (MDM)

Medical decision making (MDM) is the complexity of establishing a diagnosis and/or selecting a management option for a specific patient. It represents the thought process used by the provider to establish a diagnosis or appropriate treatment. MDM does not involve a physical examination (touching body areas of patient).

Medical decision making (MDM) includes these levels:
- Straightforward complexity
- Low complexity
- Moderate complexity
- High complexity

Each level of MDM includes 3 components, which in turn require specific elements. These are described in detail below.

For most codes, the level of service is determined by EITHER medical decision making or time. Following is a summary of the codes that include MDM and time:

Summary of E/M Codes that include Medical Decision Making (MDM)

Codes		Correct Code Determined by -		
		Medically appropriate history and/or examination	MDM	Time
99202-99205, 99212-99215	Office/other outpatient services	√	√	√
99221-99223, 99231, 99233	Hospital inpatient or observation care	√	√	√
99234-99236	Hospital inpatient or observation care services (Including admission and discharge services)	√	√	√
99242-99245, 99252-99255	Consultations	√	√	√
99282-99285	Emergency department services	√	√	
99304-99310	Nursing facility services	√	√	√
99341-99350	Home or residence services	√	√	√

Medical decision making is determined by three components:

Component Title	Component considers -
Number and complexity of problems addressed	Patient's condition(s)
Amount and/or complexity of data to be reviewed and analyzed	Data reviewed to establish a diagnosis or appropriate treatment
Risk of complications and/or morbidity and/or mortality of patient management	Patient's risk from current or possible future treatment. Includes treatment considered by not provided.

These three components, considered together, determine the level of MDM as follows:

Elements Used to Select Level of Medical Decision Making

Level of MDM	Components		
	Number and complexity of problems addressed	Amount and/or complexity of data to be reviewed and analyzed	Risk of complications and/or morbidity or mortality of patient management
Straightforward	Minimal	Minimal or none	Minimal
Low	Limited	Limited	Low
Moderate	Multiple	Moderate	Moderate
High	Extensive	Extensive	High

Each of the levels of MDM and their components are further defined. See Table 1: Levels of Medical Decision Making (MDM) in the CPT book. This describes the different levels (straightforward, low, moderate and high) and requirements for each component.

Examples in Table 1 may be more or less applicable to specific settings of care. For example:
- A decision to hospitalize a patient applies to outpatient or nursing facility encounters, whereas
- A decision to escalate a patient's hospital level of care (eg, inpatient transferred to ICU) applies to inpatient or observation encounters.

Different categories of codes have different requirements for MDM. See chapters 2-17 for details.

Each of these components and the elements that make up the component are described on the following pages.

First Component of MDM –
Number and complexity of problems addressed at the encounter

This component of medical decision making considers the severity of a patient's condition and the number of problems being addressed during the visit. Following are definitions of terms and guidelines used with this component.

Terms and Guidelines - Number and Complexity of Problems Addressed
Problem: A disease, condition, illness, injury, symptom, sign, finding, complaint or other matter addressed at the encounter. A definitive diagnosis may or may not be established at the time of the encounter.
Problem addressed: Problem evaluated or treated during the encounter by the provider who is reporting the service. Includes: • Considering possible additional testing or treatment that may ultimately not be performed due to risk/benefit analysis or choice of patient/parent/guardian/surrogate. • For hospital inpatient and observation care services, the problem addressed is the problem status on the date of the encounter. This may be significantly different than the problem's status at the time of admission. The problem may or may not be why the patient was originally admitted or why they continue to receive inpatient/observation care. Does **NOT** include: • Noting in the patient's medical record that another provider is managing the problem. The provider reporting the service is not providing any assessment, care coordination or other care for this problem; therefore it is not considered "addressed." • Referring the patient to another provider. The provider reporting the service does not evaluate (by history, examination, or diagnostic study[ies]) or consider treatment for this problem but is only referring the patient to another individual.
Presenting symptoms: Symptoms may "drive" the level of MDM if they are likely to represent a highly morbid condition. • This may apply even when the ultimate diagnosis is not highly morbid. • Evaluation and/or treatment should be consistent with the <u>likely</u> nature of the condition regardless of the final diagnosis. For example, a provider may evaluate a patient with chest pain. The final diagnosis may be muscle strain, but it could have been a heart attack. Therefore an extensive MDM is justified.
Comorbidities and underlying diseases: These conditions are not considered in selecting a level of service unless the conditions: • Are addressed. • Increase the amount and/or complexity of data to be reviewed and analyzed. • Increase the risk of complications and/or morbidity or mortality of patient management.

(continued on next page)

Terms and Guidelines - Number and Complexity of Problems Addressed (continued)
Multiple problems: Problems that by themselves have a lower severity may, when considered together, create higher risk due to their interaction.
Final diagnosis: This does not, in and of itself, determine the complexity or risk. An extensive evaluation may be required to conclude that the patient's signs or symptoms do not represent a highly morbid condition. See discussion of chest pain on previous page under Presenting Symptoms.

The level of this component is determined by the number of problems documented and the description of illness/problem as:

- Chronic
- Acute/self-limited or minor problem

Each of these is discussed in the following pages.

Number and Complexity of Problems Addressed (continued)
CHRONIC ILLNESSES/INJURIES

Level of severity for this component of MDM	Condition Stable or unstable?	Description
1 illness – Low 2 or more illnesses - Moderate	Stable	Patient is meeting the specific treatment goals.
1 or more illness – Moderate	Unstable	Condition is acutely worsening, poorly controlled with: • Exacerbation • Progression, or • Side effects of treatment. Treatment provided: • To control progression • Requires additional supportive care or treatment for side effects.
1 or more illness – High	Unstable	Condition with: • Severe exacerbation • Progression or • Side effects of treatment. Condition poses a significant risk of morbidity. May require escalation in level of care.
1 illness or injury – High	Unstable	Condition with: • Severe exacerbation • Progression or • Side effects of treatment. Condition poses a threat to life or bodily function in the near term without treatment. Symptoms may indicate a condition that is significantly probable. The probable condition would pose a potential threat to life or bodily function. The evaluation and treatment are consistent with this potential threat to life or bodily function. It is not necessary that a life-threatening condition to be the final diagnosis; only that it was indicated by the symptoms.

A decision tree on page 28 describes coding for this component of MDM for a condition designated as chronic.

24

Number and Complexity of Problems Addressed
ACUTE, SELF-LIMITED OR MINOR ILLNESSES/INJURIES

Levels for this component of MDM	Complicated/ uncomplicated or stable?	Description
Straightforward	Uncomplicated	• One self-limited or minor problem
Low – 1 illness or injury OR 2 or more self-limited or minor problems	Uncomplicated	• Two or more self-limited or minor problems OR • Risk of <u>morbidity</u> with treatment – Low • Risk of <u>mortality</u> with treatment - Little or none • Full recovery expected without functional impairment. • May be a problem that is normally self-limited or minor (Straightforward) but in this case it is not responding to a definite and prescribed course of treatment. • Treatment may require care in a hospital inpatient/ observation level setting.
Low – 1 illness	Stable	Patient is improving with treatment and, while resolution may not be complete, patient is stable with respect to this condition.
Moderate - 1 illness	Complicated	• 1 undiagnosed problem with uncertain prognosis • Illness causes systemic symptoms • Risk of <u>morbidity</u> without treatment is high • Systemic symptoms may not be general but may be a single system. Sometimes systemic general symptoms (fever, body aches, or fatigue) in a minor illness may be treated to alleviate symptoms. In this case, see self-limited or minor problem or acute, uncomplicated illness or injury.
Moderate – 1 injury	Complicated	One or more of these apply: • Treatment includes evaluation of body systems that are not directly part of the injured organ. • Injury is extensive. • Includes multiple treatment options associated with risk of morbidity.
High - 1 or more illnesses	Complicated	Condition with: • Severe exacerbation • Progression or • Side effects of treatment. Condition poses a threat to life or bodily function in the near term without treatment. Condition may include symptoms that: • Indicate a condition that is significantly probable and poses a potential threat to life or bodily function. • Require this level of evaluation/treatment because likely condition poses high level of severity. The evaluation and treatment are consistent this potential threat to life or bodily function. It is not necessary that a life-threatening condition is the final diagnosis; only that it was indicated by the symptoms.

A decision tree on page 26 describes coding for this component of MDM for a condition designated as acute, self-limited or minor.

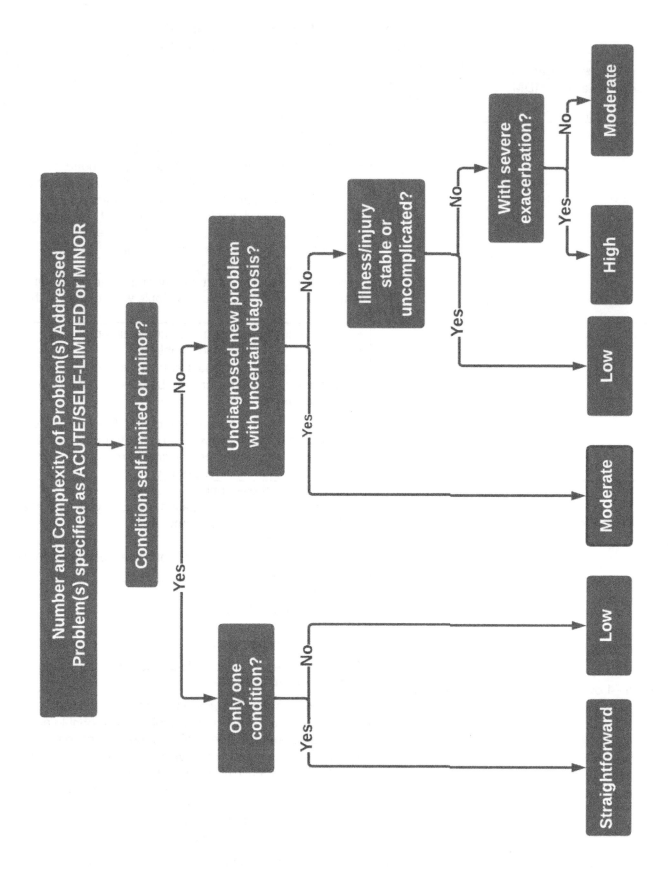

Number and Complexity of Problem(s) Addressed
Problem(s) specified as ACUTE/SELF-LIMITED or MINOR

Condition self-limited or minor?

- No → Undiagnosed new problem with uncertain diagnosis?
  - No → Illness/injury stable or uncomplicated?
    - No → With severe exacerbation?
      - No → Moderate
      - Yes → High
    - Yes → Low
  - Yes → Moderate
- Yes → Only one condition?
  - No → Low
  - Yes → Straightforward

26

Number and Complexity of Problems Address at the Encounter
Condition Specified as ACUTE/SELF-LIMITED or MINOR – Definitions

Acute – A recent or short-term problem.

Minimal problem: A problem that may not require the presence of the physician or other qualified health care professional. The service is provided under the physician's or other qualified health care professional's supervision (see 99211, 99281). Problem is self-limited or minor.

Self-limited or minor problem: A problem that runs a definite and prescribed course, is transient in nature, and is not likely to permanently alter health status.

Undiagnosed new problem with uncertain prognosis: A problem listed in a differential diagnosis that represents a condition likely to result in a high risk of morbidity without treatment.

Stable, acute illness: A problem that is new or recent for which treatment has been initiated. The patient is improved and, while resolution may not be complete, the condition is considered stable.

Unstable acute illness - Patient is not meeting their treatment goal. Condition may not have changed since patient last seen, but there is no short-term threat to life or function. The risk of morbidity without treatment is significant.

Complicated – A secondary disease or condition is aggravating an already existing one. May be caused by a procedure or treatment.

Uncomplicated – Patient has a primary illness or condition but no secondary disease or condition that makes treatment more difficult.

Acute, uncomplicated illness or injury: A recent or new short-term problem with low risk of morbidity for possible treatments. There is little to no risk of mortality with treatment, and full recovery without functional impairment is expected. A problem that is normally self-limited or minor but is not resolving consistent with a definite and prescribed course is an acute, uncomplicated illness. The treatment may or may not require care in a hospital inpatient or observation level setting.

Acute illness with systemic symptoms: An illness that causes systemic symptoms and has a high risk of morbidity without treatment. Systemic symptoms may either be general or involve a single system. For a minor illness with general systemic symptoms, such as fever, body aches, or fatigue, that may be treated to alleviate symptoms, see self-limited or minor problem or acute, uncomplicated illness or injury.

Acute, complicated injury: An injury which requires treatment that includes evaluation of body systems that are not directly part of the injured organ. The injury is extensive, or the treatment options are multiple and/or associated with risk of morbidity.

Acute illness or injury that poses a threat to life or bodily function: An acute illness that includes: 1) systemic symptoms; 2) an acute complicated injury; and/or 3) a threat to life or bodily function in the near term without treatment. Some symptoms may represent a condition that is significantly probable and poses a potential threat to life or bodily function. These may be included in this category when the evaluation and treatment are consistent with this degree of potential severity. This is a high level of complexity.

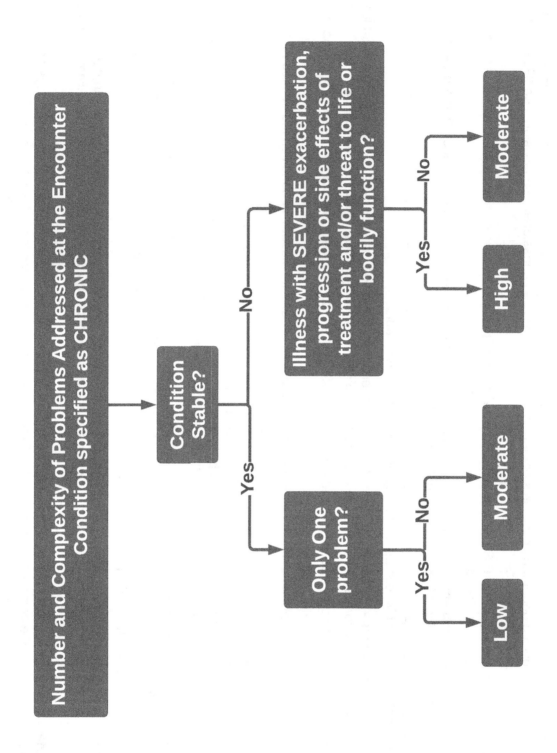

Number and Complexity of Problems Addressed at the Encounter
Condition specified as CHRONIC

- Condition Stable?
  - **No** → Illness with SEVERE exacerbation, progression or side effects of treatment and/or threat to life or bodily function?
    - **No** → Moderate
    - **Yes** → High
  - **Yes** → Only One problem?
    - **No** → Moderate
    - **Yes** → Low

Number and Complexity of Problems Addressed at the Encounter
Condition Specified as CHRONIC – Definitions

Chronic illness: A problem with an expected duration of at least one year or until the death of the patient. Conditions are treated as chronic whether or not stage or severity changes over time (eg, uncontrolled diabetes and controlled diabetes are a single chronic condition).

Stable chronic illness: Patient is meeting the specific treatment goals.

Unstable chronic illness: Patient is not meeting their treatment goal. Condition may not have changed since previous encounter. The risk of morbidity **without** treatment is significant.

Chronic illness with exacerbation, progression, or side effects of treatment: A chronic illness that is acutely worsening, poorly controlled, or progressing. Treatment is provided to control progression and requires additional supportive care or treatment for side effects.

Chronic illness with severe exacerbation, progression, or side effects of treatment: The severe exacerbation or progression of a chronic illness or severe side effects of treatment that have significant risk of morbidity and may require escalation in level of care.

Chronic illness or injury that poses a threat to life or bodily function: A chronic illness or injury with exacerbation and/or progression or side effects of treatment that poses a threat to life or bodily function in the near term without treatment.

Some symptoms may represent a condition that is significantly probable and poses a potential threat to life or bodily function. These may be considered chronic illness or injury that poses a threat to life or body function when the evaluation and treatment are consistent with this degree of potential severity.

Second Component of MDM –
Amount and/or Complexity of Data to be Reviewed and Analyzed

This component of medical decision making considers the amount and/or complexity of data that must be obtained, ordered, reviewed and analyzed in order for the provider to select a diagnose or treatment option for the patient. See page 34 for the categories used with this component.

The level of this component depends on whether: data were gathered from another source (another provider or independent historian); or from a test ordered/performed/reviewed by the provider reporting the service; or by the provider discussed test results with another provider.

Terms and Guidelines – Amount and/or Complexity of Data to be Reviewed and Analyzed
Definition of Terms/Guidelines
Data: Medical records, tests, and/or other information that must be obtained, ordered, reviewed, and analyzed to diagnose or treat a patient. Includes: • Information obtained from multiple sources. • Communications from other providers that are not reported separately using another code. • Interpretation of tests that are not reported separately using another code. If little or no data is reviewed, use the straightforward level of this element. See page 33 for a comparison of different sources of data (external, unique, appropriate).
Analyzed: The process of using the data as part of the MDM. The data itself may not be subject to analysis (eg, glucose level), but it is still part of the provider's thought processes to diagnose, evaluate, or treat this patient. Data analysis is **NOT** included in this component if it is part of a service with a separately reported professional component. For example: • A pregnant patient is seen in the emergency department and an ultrasound is performed. The ultrasound is reviewed by her obstetrician in a subsequent encounter. • The obstetrician reports the ultrasound code with a modifier 26 (professional component). • The analysis of the ultrasound is **NOT** included in the MDM for the encounter since it is already reported using the ultrasound code.
Combination of data elements: A combination of different data elements can be added together for this component. For example, notes reviewed, tests ordered, tests reviewed, or independent historian. These elements can be added together. For example: • Count each element separately: A unique test ordered, plus an unrelated note reviewed and information obtained from an independent historian. Count as 3 elements. • Count as one test: One test, ordered and then reviewed. Count either the ordering or the review/analysis, but not both.

(continued on next page)

Terms and Guidelines – Amount and/or Complexity of Data
Terms and Guidelines – Amount and/or Complexity of Data to be Reviewed and Analyzed (continued)
Data Elements by Category

Independent interpretation – Part of these categories:
Category 1 - Moderate or high levels of MDM
Category 2 - Low level of MDM

The provider interprets the results of a test.

An interpretation should be documented. Documentation does not need to include a complete report for the test.

Interpretation does **NOT** include a simple review of the results. However, if the provider interprets the results, which involves additional work, then count separately both an order and interpretation for the test.

Tests - Part of these categories:
Category 1 - Review and ordering of tests
Category 2 - Interpretation of tests for moderate and high levels of MDM

Tests are imaging, laboratory psychometric, or physiologic data.

- A clinical laboratory panel (eg, basic metabolic panel [80047]) is a single test.
- The difference between single or multiple tests is defined using the CPT code set (one code = one test).
- A test may be reviewed but no independent interpretation is required. Count this is a review but not an interpretation.

Ordering tests:
- Tests ordered are considered analyzed when the results are reported.
- A test may be normally performed for this condition but is considered too risky for this patient; therefore, the test was not done. This counts as a test since it was considered.
- Tests ordered during an encounter are counted for that encounter.
- Tests ordered outside of an encounter are counted during the encounter in which the results are analyzed.

Recurring order for a test:
- Each new test result is counted separately during the encounter in which it is analyzed.
- An encounter that includes an order for monthly prothrombin times is counted as one prothrombin time ordered and reviewed each month.
- Analysis of additional results during a subsequent encounter is counted again as a single test.

Unique test: Count as one test:
- Multiple results from the same unique test (eg, serial blood glucose values) compared during an E/M service.
- Tests that have overlapping elements, even if they are identified with distinct CPT codes. For example, a CBC with differential include these tests: hemoglobin test, CBC without differential, and platelet count.

Tests do **NOT** include:
- Pulse oximetry
- Tests included in another CPT code

(continued on next page)

Terms and Guidelines – Amount and/or Complexity of Data to be Reviewed and Analyzed (continued)

Data Elements by Category

Discussion – Part of this category:

Category 3 – Moderate or high levels of MDM

A discussion requires a direct, interactive exchange of information or data.

The discussion:
- Does **NOT** need to be on the date of the encounter.
- Is counted only once and only when it is used in the decision making for the encounter.
- May be asynchronous (communication using electronic means or other messaging, but not at the same moment).
- Must be initiated and completed within a short time period (eg, within a day or two).
- Must be from an appropriate source. See definition of appropriate source on next page.

The discussion does **NOT** include:
- Discussions with family or informal caregivers.
- Sending chart notes or written exchanges that are part of progress notes.
- Exchange of information through intermediaries (eg, one provider relays information through clinical staff or trainees to other provider).

Independent historian - Part of these categories:

Category 1 - Moderate and high level of MDM

Category 2 – Low level of MDM

An individual (eg, parent, guardian, surrogate, spouse, witness) who provides a history in addition to a history provided by the patient.

The independent history does **NOT** need to be obtained in person but must be obtained directly from the historian providing the information, not through a third party.

An independent history may be necessary because:
- The patient is unable to provide a complete or reliable history (eg, due to developmental stage, dementia, or psychosis) OR
- The provider judges that a confirmatory history is necessary OR
- There is a conflict or poor communication between multiple historians and more than one historian is needed.

Does **NOT** include:
- Translation services

See page 34 for a complete list of components for each category.

The definitions for sources of data used in these categories of amount and/or complexity of data include similar, overlapping terms. These are as follows:

Comparison of Sources of Data

Term	Definition
External source/ physician or other QHP	A provider who is **NOT** in the same group as the reporting provider or Is of a different specialty or subspecialty in the same group
Appropriate source	An external source May include nonphysician providers involved in management of patient Examples: lawyer, parole officer, case manager, teacher Does **NOT** include discussions with patient or family
Unique source	An external source Data may come from a provider or a facility All materials from a unique source are counted as one element within the data component of MDM

33

The levels for this component of MDM (amount and/or complexity of data) include 3 possible categories, but the requirements within each category are not the same for low, moderate and high levels.

The level for this component is determined by the data in these categories:

Amount and/or Complexity of Data to be Reviewed and Analyzed (continued)		
Levels for this component of MDM	**Data Required**	**Description**
Straightforward	Minimal or none	No categories required.
Low	Limited	Must include at least 1 of these 2 categories - **Category 1:** Tests and Documents At least 2 of these 3 bullets within this category are required: • Review of prior external note(s) from each unique source. • Review of the result(s) of each unique test • Ordering of each unique test. **Category 2:** Assessment requiring an independent historian(s)
Moderate	Moderate	Must include at least 1 out of these 3 categories - **Category 1:** Tests, documents or independent historian At least 3 of these 4 bullets within this category are required: • Review of prior external note(s) from each unique source. • Review of the result(s) of each unique test. • Ordering of each unique test. • Assessment requiring an independent historian(s). **Category 2:** Independent interpretation of tests • Interpretation of a test performed by this or another provider (not separately reported). **Category 3:** Discussion of management or test interpretation • Discussion with external provider (not separately reported).
High	Extensive	Must include at least 2 out of these 3 categories – **Category 1:** Tests, documents or independent historian At least 3 of these 4 bullets within this category are required: • Review of prior external note(s) from each unique source. • Review of the result(s) of each unique test. • Ordering of each unique test. • Assessment requiring an independent historian(s). **Category 2:** Independent interpretation of tests • Interpretation of a test performed by this or another provider (not separately reported). **Category 3:** Discussion of management or test interpretation • Discussion with external provider (not separately reported).

Note that the definition of categories 1 and 2 are different for low level and moderate/high levels of this component (amount and/or complexity of data) of MDM.

Independent historian is included in Category 2 for low level while it is included in Category 1 for moderate and high levels.

In addition, the requirements for these levels are different.
- The **LOW** level of this component requires documentation of **EITHER** Category 1 (2 bullets) or Category 2. The level can be used if only one of these categories is documented. Category 3 is not used for this level.
- The **MODERATE** level of this component requires documentation of **EITHER** Category 1 (3 bullets), Category 2 or Category 3. This level can be used if any one of these 3 categories is documented.
- The **HIGH** level of this component requires documentation of **ANY 2** of these three categories. If using category 2, must include 3 bullets. This level can be used only if 2 categories are documented.

A decision tree on the next page describes coding for this component.

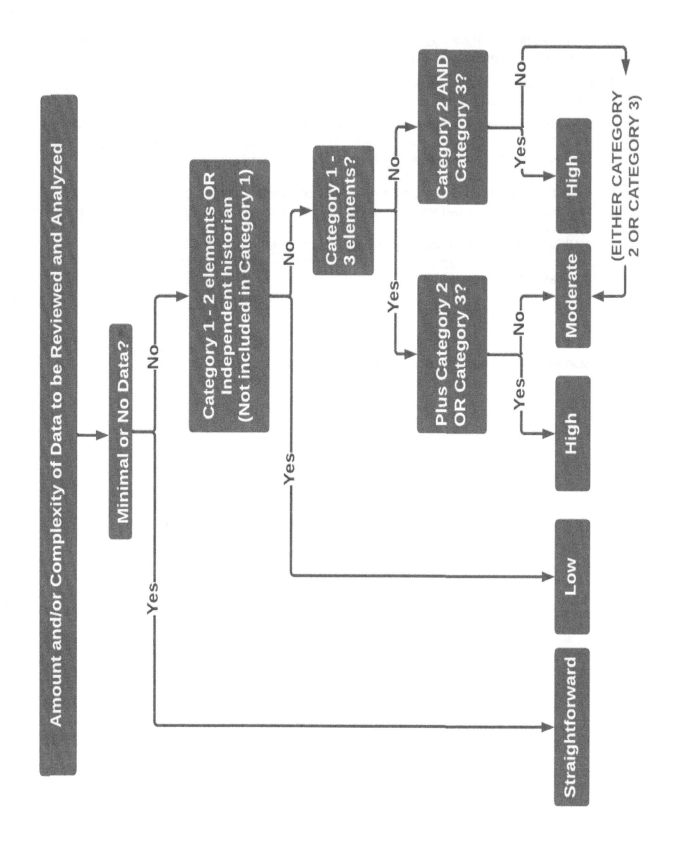

Amount and/or Complexity of Data to be Reviewed - Definitions

For Low level of this element:

<u>Category 1</u> - Tests and Documents. This category includes these elements:

- Review of prior external note(s) from each unique source
- Review of the result(s) of each unique test
- Ordering of each unique test

<u>Category 2</u> - Assessment Requiring an Independent Historian(s).

At least 2 of these 3 elements are required in order to meet the requirements for low level.

<u>Category 3</u> is not included in low level.

For Moderate and High levels of this element:

<u>Category 1</u> - Tests, Documents or Independent Historian. (Note addition of Independent Historian in category title, which was not included in low level). This category includes these elements:

- Review of prior external note(s) from each unique source
- Review of the result(s) of each unique test
- Ordering of each unique test
- Assessment requiring an independent historian(s)

At least 3 of the elements listed above are required in order to meet the requirements of moderate or high of this component.

<u>Category 2</u> - Independent Interpretation of Tests. (Note that this title is different than the category title for low level).

<u>Category 3</u> - Discussion of Management or Test Interpretation and includes discussion with external physician/other qualified health care professional/appropriate source (not separately reported).

Moderate level requires documentation of at least one category: Category 1 (3 elements), Category 2 OR Category 3.

High level requires documentation of 3 elements from at least 2 categories: Category 1 (3 elements) OR Category 2 OR Category 3.

Third Component of MDM –
Risk of Complications and/or Morbidity or Mortality of Patient Management

This component of medical decision making considers the risk of complications from the possible <u>diagnostic procedures and treatments</u> provided to the patient, **NOT** from the patient's <u>problem or condition</u>. Risks arising from the problem are captured in the first component (problem addressed) of Medical Decision Making.

Terms and Guidelines – Risk of Complications and/or Morbidity or Mortality of Patient Management
Risk: The probability and/or consequences rising from a provider's management (treatment or diagnostic testing) of a condition. Risk is not strictly defined. Definitions of risk are based on: • The usual behavior and thought processes of a physician or other qualified health care professional in the same specialty. • The common meanings that providers use for terms such as high, medium, low, or minimal risk. Quantification (counting) is not required for these definitions. • Quantification may be used when evidence-based medicine has established probabilities. The level of risk is affected by the possible adverse effects that might result from management of the patient, not from the patient's condition. For example: • A low probability of death may have a high risk of adverse effects from treatment. For example, a provider may consider prescribing a medication with a low potential for causing the patient's death but a high risk of causing fatigue, an adverse effect. • A high probability of a minor, self-limited adverse effect from treatment may be low risk. For example, a provider may consider prescribing diuretics with a high potential for increasing patient's urination but low risk of causing complications.
Management options: Possible choices considered by the provider for diagnosis and treatment for a patient. Risk includes possible management options selected and those options that were considered but not selected. The provider may discuss risks and benefits of each management option with the patient and/or family. In selecting a final management option, the provider considers patient and/or family preferences and any patient and/or family education that will be needed. A decision about hospitalization includes consideration of alternative levels of care that may or may not be appropriate in a specific case. For example: • Provider considers hospitalization of a psychiatric patient. However, the patient has a sufficient degree of support from others living in their residence and therefore does not require hospitalization. • Provider considers admission to inpatient care for a patient with advanced dementia and other acute conditions. However, this patient is receiving palliative treatment, so hospitalization would not be appropriate.
Morbidity: A state of illness or functional impairment resulting from patient management that is expected to be of substantial duration during which: • Function is limited • Quality of life is impaired, OR • Organ damage occurs that may not be transient despite treatment.

(continued on next page)

Mortality: A state of illness or functional impairment resulting from patient management that may result in death of the patient.

Drug therapy requiring intensive monitoring for toxicity: Monitoring of a drug, being administered to a patient, that has the potential to cause serious morbidity or death. This element represents a high level of MDM.

Monitoring impacts the possible management options for a patient's condition (eg, if there is an adverse effect found, other less toxic options will be considered). Monitoring includes:

- Assessment primarily for presence/absence of adverse effects, **NOT f**or whether or not the drug is working as desired in treating the condition.
- Either generally accepted monitoring applicable for all patients or patient-specific monitoring.
- Either long-term or short-term assessment. Must be performed at least quarterly.
- Laboratory tests, physiologic tests or imaging.

Examples:

- Monitoring for cytopenia in use of antineoplastic agent between dose cycles OR
- Intensive monitoring of electrolytes in a patient who is undergoing chemotherapy.

This element does **NOT** include:

- Monitoring glucose levels during insulin therapy (because the monitoring is to evaluate the therapeutic effect of the insulin, not the drug's toxicity).
- Annual monitoring of electrolytes and renal function for a patient on a diuretic (because it is not performed quarterly).
- Monitoring using history or examination.

The levels of this component of MDM are determined by the risk of complications, morbidity or mortality.

Risk of Complications and/or Morbidity or Mortality of Patient Management (continued)

Levels of this component of MDM	Amount of Risk	Description
Straightforward	Minimal or none	Minimal risk of morbidity from additional diagnostic testing or treatment.
Low	Limited	Low risk of morbidity from additional diagnostic testing or treatment.
Moderate	Moderate	Moderate risk of morbidity from diagnostic testing or treatment. Examples: • Prescription drug management. • Decision regarding minor surgery with identified patient or procedure risk factors. • Decision regarding elective major surgery without identified patient or procedure risk factors. • Diagnosis or treatment significantly limited by social determinants of health.
High	Extensive	High risk of morbidity from additional diagnostic testing or treatment. Examples: • Drug therapy requiring intensive monitoring for toxicity. • Decision regarding elective major surgery with identified patient or procedure risk factors. • Decision regarding emergency major surgery. • Decision regarding hospitalization or escalation of hospital-level care. • Decision not to resuscitate or to de-escalate care because of poor prognosis. • Decision regarding parenteral controlled substances.

Note: Moderate and high levels of this component are defined only using examples, not a definition.

Minor, elective or major surgery may be considered, but may ultimately not be performed. The consideration of the surgery counts for this component.

Different categories of E/M codes have different requirements. See chapters 2-17.

On the next page is a comparison of the components of high risk and moderate risk.

Comparison – Elements within Moderate and High Risk Medical Decision Making

High risk and moderate risk have some similar elements. These are compared below.

Risk from -	Moderate MDM	High MDM
Medications	Prescription drug management	Drug therapy requiring intensive monitoring for toxicity
Surgery	Minor surgery with identified patient or procedure risk factors	
	Elective major surgery without identified patient or procedure risk factors	Elective major surgery with identified patient or procedure risk factors
		Emergency major surgery
Other risk categories	Diagnosis or treatment significantly limited by social determinants of health (SDOH)	
		Decision regarding hospitalization or escalation of hospital-level care
		Decision not to resuscitate or to de-escalate care because of poor prognosis
		Parenteral controlled substances

If the documentation indicates that the encounter includes elements that are listed for moderate and high levels, use the higher level. For example, a patient may have treatment that is significantly limited by social determinants of health (moderate level of risk), but also had emergency major surgery (high level of risk). This is considered a high level of risk.

A decision tree on the next page describes coding for this element.

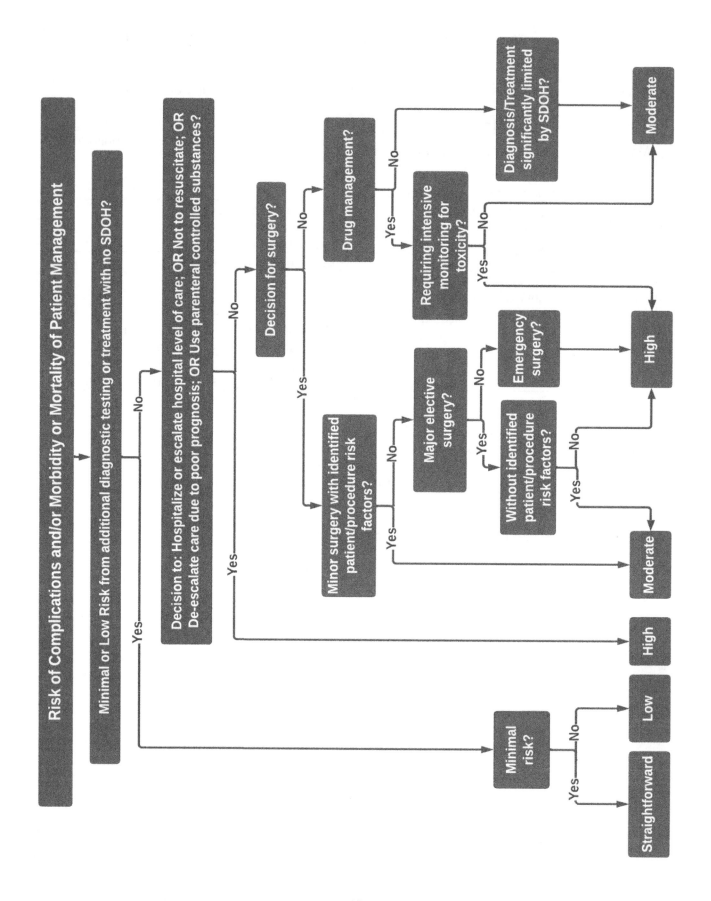

Risk of Complications and/or Morbidity or Mortality of Patient Management

Minimal or Low Risk from additional diagnostic testing or treatment with no SDOH?

- No →
  - **Decision to: Hospitalize or escalate hospital level of care; OR De-escalate care due to poor prognosis; OR Not to resuscitate; OR Use parenteral controlled substances?**
    - Yes → **High**
    - No →
      - **Decision for surgery?**
        - Yes →
          - **Minor surgery with identified patient/procedure risk factors?**
            - Yes → **Moderate**
            - No →
              - **Major elective surgery?**
                - Yes →
                  - **Without identified patient/procedure risk factors?**
                    - Yes → **Moderate**
                    - No → **High**
                - No →
                  - **Emergency surgery?** → **High**
        - No →
          - **Drug management?**
            - Yes →
              - **Requiring intensive monitoring for toxicity?**
                - Yes → **High**
                - No → **Moderate**
            - No →
              - **Diagnosis/Treatment significantly limited by SDOH?** → **Moderate**
- Yes →
  - **Minimal risk?**
    - Yes → **Straightforward**
    - No → **Low**

The Risk of Complications and/or Morbidity or Mortality of Patient Management

Surgery—Minor or Major: The classification of surgery into minor or major is based on the common meaning of such terms when used by trained clinicians. These terms are not the same as those used in the global surgical package, described on page 203.

Surgery—Elective or Emergency: Elective procedures and emergent or urgent procedures describe the timing of a procedure. An elective procedure is typically planned in advance (eg, scheduled for weeks later). An emergent procedure is typically performed immediately or with minimal delay to allow for patient stabilization. Both elective and emergent procedures may be minor or major procedures.

Surgery—Risk Factors, Patient or Procedure: Risk factors are those that are relevant both to the patient and the procedure. Evidence-based risk calculators may be used, but are not required, in assessing patient and procedure risk.

Morbidity: A state of illness or functional impairment that is expected to be of substantial duration during which function is limited, quality of life is impaired, or there is organ damage that may not be transient despite treatment.

Drug therapy requiring intensive monitoring for toxicity:

- The drug (therapeutic agent): Requires intensive monitoring because it has the potential to cause serious morbidity or death.
- The monitoring: Performed for assessment of adverse effects and not primarily for assessment of therapeutic efficacy (whether or not the drug is effective). The monitoring:
  - Should follow generally accepted practice for the agent but may be patient-specific in some cases.
  - Affects the level of MDM in an encounter in the monitoring is considered (not necessarily provided) in the management of the patient.
  - May be long-term or short-term. Monitoring must be at least quarterly. The monitoring may be performed with a laboratory test, a physiologic test, or imaging.
  - May be monitoring for cytopenia in the use of an antineoplastic agent between dose cycles.

- Monitoring does **NOT** include:
  - Monitoring by history or examination
  - Monitoring glucose levels during insulin therapy. The primary reason for the monitoring is to evaluate the therapeutic effect of the drug (unless severe hypoglycemia is a current, significant concern), not toxicity of the drug.
  - Annual electrolytes and renal function for a patient on a diuretic. The frequency does not meet the threshold of quarterly.

Social determinants of health (SDOH): Economic and social conditions that influence the health of people and communities. Examples may include food or housing insecurity or living alone.

Parenteral controlled substances: Schedule I-V drugs (such as heroin, methadone, Xanax) administered/given by a route other than the alimentary canal (subcutaneous, intramuscular, intravenous, intra-arterial, or intradermal).

43

Using the Three Components to Determine the Level of Medical Decision Making (MDM)

To determine the level of MDM, first determine the elements within each of the three components. Then, find which level of the component is represented by these elements. Finally, use the level of all three components to determine the final level of MDM.

Following is an example of determining level of MDM:

Level of Medical Decision Making	Components of MDM		
	1 Number/Complexity of Problems Addressed	2 Amount and/or Complexity of Data Reviewed and Analyzed	3 Risk of Complications of Patient Management
Minimal			
Low	Two self-limited or minor problems	Category 1: ordering of a test; review of results of a test	
Moderate			Prescription drug management
High			

In this example, the final level of MDM is low since the criteria for components one and two were met. It does not matter that the third component (risk) is at a higher, moderate level. See Appendix A, example 1.

If each component is a different level, use the level of MDM in the middle. For example:

Level of Medical Decision Making	Components of MDM		
	1 Number/Complexity of Problems Addressed	2 Amount and/or Complexity of Data Reviewed and Analyzed	3 Risk of Complications of Patient Management
Minimal	Two self-limited or minor problems		
Low		Category 1: ordering of a test; review of results of a test	
Moderate			Prescription drug management
High			

In this example, the level of MDM is low since the criteria for component two (data) was met and the criteria for the third component (risk) was met or exceeded. The level of risk exceeds (is more than) the required level for low. The level of problems addressed is minimal. The coder may round down (from moderate to low risk) but not round up (from low to moderate complexity of data).

Selecting a Code Using Time

For many codes, the level of service is determined by EITHER medical decision making OR time. Other codes are selected only according to time. Following is a summary of these codes:

Summary of E/M Codes Reported Using Time

Codes		Correct Code Determined by -		
		Medically appropriate history and/or examination	MDM	Time
99202-99205, 99211-99215	Office/other outpatient services	√	√	√
99221-99223, 99231- 99233	Hospital inpatient or observation care	√	√	√
99234-99236	Hospital inpatient or observation care services (Including admission and discharge services)	√	√	√
99238, 99239	Hospital discharge management			√
99242-99245, 99252-99255	Consultations	√	√	√
99291, +99292	Critical care services			√
99304-99310	Nursing facility services	√	√	√
99315, 99316	Nursing facility discharge management			√
99341-99345, 99347-99350	Home or residence services	√	√	√
99358, +99359	Prolonged services on date other than face-to-face service			√
99360	Standby services			√
99366-99368	Medical team conferences			√
99374-99380	Care plan oversight services			√
99401-99404, 99406-99409, 99411, 99412	Counseling and risk factor reduction and behavioral change intervention			√
+99415, +99416	Prolonged clinical staff services			√
+99417, +99418	Prolonged outpatient services on same date as other E/M service			√
99421-99423	Online digital E/M services			√
99424-99427	Principal care management services			√
99441-99443	Telephone services			√

(Continued on next page)

Summary of E/M Codes Reported Using Time (continued)

Codes		Correct Code Determined by -		
		Medically appropriate history and/or examination	MDM	Time
99446-99452	Interprofessional telephone/ internet/electronic health record consultations			√
99453, 99454, 99091, 99473, 99474	Digitally stored data service/remote physiologic monitoring			√
99457, +99458	Remote physiologic monitoring treatment management services			√
99466, +99467, 99485, +99486	Pediatric critical care patient transport			√
99487-+99489	Complex chronic care management services			√
99490, 99491, +99437, +99439	Chronic care management services			√
99492, 99493, +99494	Psychiatric collaborative care management services			√
99497, +99498	Advance care planning			√

Guidelines – Selecting a Code Using Time (continued)

Calculating Time

Each code that may be reported using time has a required time threshold. This threshold must be met in order to report the code; you can **NOT** round up to report the next highest level.

For example, a service that is documented as 25 minutes must be reported using code 99202 (with a time threshold of 15 minutes). The coder can **NOT** round up to code 99203 (with a time threshold of 30 minutes).

The exception to this threshold requirement is code 99483 (cognitive assessment and care plan services), which lists a typical time, not a specific time which must be met.

Time may be spent:
- In a face-to-face encounter with the provider and patient and/or family/caregiver.
- In a non-face-to-face service personally spent by the provider on the same day as a face-to-face encounter.
- In a non-face-to-face service only.

Count time spent:
- Providing activities that require a physician or other qualified health care professional and
- In any location (eg, whether on or off the inpatient unit or in or out of the outpatient office).

Do **NOT** count time:
- Spent performing other separately reported service(s).
- Providing activities normally performed by clinical staff.
- Spent traveling to/from the patient's location.
- Teaching others when the subject matter is general and not limited to discussions required for the management of a specific patient.

Activities That May be Measured by Time

Time spent by a physician or other qualified health care professional includes the following activities, when performed:
- Face-to-face and/or non-face-to-face services.
- Preparing to see the patient (eg, review of tests).
- Obtaining and/or reviewing separately obtained history.
- Performing a medically appropriate examination and/or evaluation.
- Counseling and educating the patient/family/caregiver.
- Ordering medications, tests, or procedures.
- Referring and communicating with other health care professionals (when not separately reported).
- Documenting clinical information in the electronic or other health record.
- Independently interpreting results (when interpretation is not separately reported) and communicating results to the patient/family/caregiver.
- Coordinating care (when not separately reported using another code).

Different categories of E/M codes have different requirements for selecting a code using time. See chapters 2-17.

1. Medical decision making (MDM) is based on the:
    a. Number of diagnoses the physician must consider
    b. Patient's risk of morbidity
    c. Amount of data the physician must evaluate
    d. All of these elements are part of the MDM

2. An appropriate examination and history is determined by:
    a. Centers for Medicare and Medicaid Services
    b. The physician providing the service
    c. The medical coder
    d. Definition in the E/M guidelines

3. A provider documents two self-limited or minor problems. For the number and complexity of problems addressed component of MDM, this is:
    a. Straightforward level
    b. Low level
    c. Moderate level
    d. High level

4. A patient's condition is improving (meeting treatment goals), but not yet resolved. This condition is considered:
    a. Complicated
    b. Acute
    c. Chronic
    d. Stable
    e. Unstable

5. For the high level of amount and/or complexity of data to be reviewed and analyzed, use of an independent historian is part of:
    a. Category 1
    b. Category 2
    c. Category 3

6. An example of high risk of morbidity is:
    a. Decision for elective major surgery without identified patient or procedure risk factors
    b. Treatment significantly limited by social determinants of health
    c. Prescription drug management
    d. Drug therapy requiring intensive monitoring for toxicity

7. A provider documents this MDM: number/complexity of problems addressed – low; amount/complexity of data reviewed and analyzed – moderate; risks of management – low. The MDM for this patient is:
    a. Straightforward
    b. Low
    c. Moderate
    d. High

8. Do not count total time for:
   a. Face-to-face encounters with the provider and patient and/or family/caregiver
   b. Non-face-to-face time spent with the patient and/or family/caregiver on date of encounter
   c. Time spent by the provider traveling to patient's location
   d. Ordering medications for the patient

See Appendix B for quiz answers.

Chapter 2

CPT® Office or Other Outpatient Services

These codes are reported for outpatient services. An outpatient is an individual who has **NOT** been formally admitted to a facility as an inpatient. The setting may be physician's office, hospital clinic and other ambulatory facilities.

The broad definition of outpatient settings includes settings such as emergency department or observation care, or other types of services, such as outpatient consultation. However, these settings and types of services have their own separate sets of codes and therefore are not discussed in this chapter.

See Appendix A for a form to assist in selecting an E/M code for office and other outpatient services.

Summary of Specific Criteria Used to Select Office or Other Outpatient Codes

Services		Correct Code Determined by -		
		Medically appropriate history and/or examination	MDM	Time
99202-99205	Office/other outpatient services, new patient	√	√	√
99212-99215	Office/other outpatient services, established patient	√	√	√

Note: code 99211 is also used for office or other outpatient visits. These visits may not require the presence of a physician or other qualified healthcare professional. No medically appropriate history and/or examination, medical decision making, or total time is included in this code. This code is only used for established patients.

A new add-on code was added for Medicare patients (but may be utilized by other payers): G2211 Office and Outpatient E/M visit complexity. This code can be used regardless of the provider's specialty. It can be used when the provider is either:

- The continuing focal point for all the patient's needed services, such as a primary care practitioner.
- Providing ongoing care for a single, serious condition or a complex condition, such as sickle cell disease or HIV.

The documentation must indicate the medical necessity of the add-on code.

Code G2211 can **NOT** be used when another associated E/M service is being reported with a modifier 25.

Specific Times and MDM Levels Used for Office and Other Outpatient Codes

Codes	Code selected using EITHER time measured in minutes or medical decision making	
	Time spent on date of service	Level of medical decision making
New Patients		
99202	15 minutes	Straightforward
99203	30 minutes	Low
99204	45 minutes	Moderate
99205	60 minutes	High
Established Patients		
99211	Presence of physician not required. No time established	N/A
99212	10 minutes	Straightforward
99213	20 minutes	Low
99214	30 minutes	Moderate
99215	40 minutes	High

Guidelines – Office or Other Outpatient Services (99202-99205, 99212-99215)

GENERAL GUIDELINES
These codes are reported for outpatient services (physician's office, hospital clinic and other ambulatory facilities).
These codes are provided face-to-face with patient or using telemedicine services if appropriate.
For a consultation in this setting, use outpatient consultation codes 99242-99245.
There are separate codes for new or established patients.
There are no separate codes for initial or subsequent service.

SELECTING CODES USING TIME OR MDM
These codes are selected using time or medical decision making.
Sometimes the encounter lasts 15 minutes or longer than the time listed in the highest level within a code category. If selecting the code using time, use the highest level of E/M code and prolonged services code +99417. Code +99417 can be listed in multiple units when appropriate.

- For example, a new patient encounter lasted a total of 75 minutes. List code 99205 (60 minutes) plus +99417 (additional 15 minutes).
- See Chapter 10 for more information on prolonged services.

OTHER SERVICES
Services **NOT** included in these codes. Report separately if appropriate:

- Significant, separately reportable procedures or other services. The service must include the requirements to meet the level of an E/M service (using MDM or time).
Report two codes: an office or other outpatient E/M code and a code for the other service. Add a modifier, such as modifier 24, if appropriate, to the code for the other service.

- Patient transferred <u>from</u> office or other outpatient setting <u>to</u> hospital inpatient/observation setting.
Report two codes: one for the office setting and one for the inpatient/observation setting if the transfer was initiated by same provider. Add a modifier 25 to the outpatient E/M service to indicate a significant, separately identifiable service.

Do **NOT** report separately:
- A code for an insignificant procedure or other service. This is a service that does not meet the MDM or time requirements for an E/M code.

1. A physician sees a new patient who had received a severe beating in a mugging. He treats the wounds and counsels the patient, who is quite traumatized by the event. The physician documents straightforward medical decision making. Code 99202 has a time threshold of 15 minutes. However, the physician spent a total of 30 minutes (code 99203) with this patient because of the exam and counseling. The coder reports:
   a. Code 99202
   b. Code 99203
   c. Code 99204
   d. Code 99205

2. A physician sees an established patient. She provides moderate level of medical decision making. The encounter lasts 25 minutes. The coder reports:
   a. Code 99211
   b. Code 99212
   c. Code 99213
   d. Code 99214

3. Which of these elements are NOT used to select an outpatient code:
   a. Examination and history
   b. Time
   c. Medical decision making
   d. New or established patient

See Appendix B for quiz answers.

Chapter 3

CPT® Hospital Inpatient and Observation Care Services

These codes are reported for services provided to a patient who is either an inpatient or designated as observation status. These codes are also used for partial hospitalization services.

See Appendix A for a form to assist in selecting an E/M code using these components.

Following is a summary of the hospital inpatient and observation care codes:

Summary of Specific Criteria Used to Select Hospital Inpatient and Observation Codes

Services		Correct Code Determined by -		
		Medically appropriate history and/or examination	MDM	Time
99221-99223, 99231, 99233	Hospital inpatient or observation care	√	√	√
99234-99236	Hospital inpatient or observation care services (admit/discharge same date)	√	√	√
99238, 99239	Hospital discharge management			√

These codes are selected by minutes spent with the patient "per day." If multiple visits occur over the course of a single calendar date in the same setting, a single service is reported.

Specific Times and MDM Levels Used for Hospital/Observation Care Codes

Codes	Code selected using EITHER time or medical decision making	
	Time spent on date of service	Level of medical decision making
Initial Hospital/Observation Care		
99221	40 minutes	Straightforward or Low
99222	55 minutes	Moderate
99223	75 minutes	High
Subsequent Hospital/Observation Care		
99231	25 minutes	Straightforward or Low
99232	35 minutes	Moderate
99233	50 minutes	High
Same Day Admission/Discharge Care		
99234	45 minutes	Straightforward or Low
99235	70 minutes	Moderate
99236	85 minutes	High
Discharge Services		
99238	30 minutes or less	-
99239	More than 30 minutes	-

Guidelines – Hospital Inpatient and Observation Care Services
(99221-99223, 99231-99236, 99238, 99239)

GENERAL GUIDELINES
These codes are used to report services provided to a patient who is either an inpatient or designated as observation status. They are also used for partial hospitalization services.
A patient may be in a facility and designated as "observation status." It is not necessary that the patient be located in a specified observation area within the facility.
There are separate codes for initial or subsequent service.
For a consultation in this setting, use inpatient consultation codes 99252-99255.
There are no separate codes for new and established patients.
There are separate codes for initial and subsequent visits.

Problem Addressed During Encounter
The problem addressed is: • The problem as presented on the date of the encounter. • The problem being managed or co-managed by the reporting provider at this encounter; it may or may not be reason the patient was first admitted or remain in the facility. • May be significantly different than the problem that was present on admission.

SELECTING CODES USING TIME OR MDM
Codes 99221-99223, 99231-99236 are selected using medical decision making or time.
These are reported per day.
• **If the code is selected using MDM,** add together the MDM components over the course of the calendar date. For example, consider both the tests performed in the morning and those performed later in the same day.
• **If the code is selected using time,** sum the time over the course of the day.
Total time may or may not be continuous.
If more than one E/M service is being reported, count only the time spent providing the individual service. No time may be counted twice.
A continuous service that spans two calendar dates is a coded as a single service. Use a single code, and report the code on one calendar date.
The encounter may last longer 15 minutes longer than the time listed in the highest level within a code category (initial service [75 minutes], subsequent service [50 minutes] or same date admit and discharge [85 minutes]). Use prolonged services code +99418. Code +99418 can be listed in multiple units if appropriate. • For example, an initial inpatient encounter lasted a total of 90 minutes. List code 99223 (75 minutes) plus +99218 (additional 15 minutes). • See Chapter 10 for more information on prolonged services.
Codes 99238, 99239 are selected using time in minutes only.

(continued on next page)

ENCOUNTERS

Initial Visits (99221-99223)

Initial care codes 99221-99223 are reported for services face-to-face with patient.

These codes are reported once per patient per admission.

Use these codes when patient has **NOT** received any professional services from this provider or another provider of the exact same specialty and subspecialty who belongs to the same group practice during this stay.

An advanced practice nurse or physician assistant may work with the provider. They are considered as working in the exact same specialty and subspecialty as the provider. Only one or the other may report an initial admission service.

The patient may have received services from this provider during a previous stay or encounter.

Subsequent Visits (99231-99233)

Subsequent care codes 99231-99233 can be reported for face-to-face services or telemedicine services if appropriate.

Admission/Discharge on SAME Date (99234-99236)

Use these codes for patients who were admitted and discharged on the same date.

The admission and discharge must be provided by the same individual.

The stay must be more than eight hours.

These codes are reported using time or medical decision making.

The care must include at least these two encounters on the same date:
- One encounter for the initial admission to hospital/observation care.
- Other encounter for discharge services.

Do **NOT** use these codes:
- If the two encounters listed above are not documented. Use codes for an initial care code (99221-99223) only.
- If time of the encounter is 8 hours or less. Use codes for an initial care only.
- With discharge services codes 99238 and 99239.

Do **NOT** count time spent providing other service in time spent providing discharge services.

(continued on next page)

ENCOUNTERS (continued)

Admission/Discharge on DIFFERENT Dates (99238, 99239)

Use these codes for patients who were admitted and discharged on different dates.

These codes are used with initial or subsequent inpatient/observation care codes.

These codes are reported using time only. Time may or may not be continuous.

Discharge services are provided by:
- The physician or other qualified health care professional who is responsible for discharge services. Report discharge codes 99238, 99239.
- Other providers may give instructions to the patient and/or family/caregiver and coordinate post-discharge services. Report these codes for subsequent inpatient/observation care.

Discharge services include, as appropriate:
- Final examination of the patient.
- Discussion of the hospital stay.
- Instructions for continuing care to all relevant caregivers.
- Preparation of discharge records, prescriptions, and referral forms.

Do **NOT** report 99328, 99239 with codes for same day admission and discharge (99221-99223)

MULTIPLE SETTINGS – SAME PROVIDER

Transfer from Another Site to Hospital Inpatient/Observation Care

Patient transferred from another site to hospital inpatient/observation by same provider. The other site may be a hospital emergency department, office, or nursing facility.

- List two codes: one code for services provided in the initial (other) site with a modifier 25; and a hospital/observation care code.

If reporting two codes and a prolonged services code, use the prolonged services code related to the primary service reported, regardless of the patient's location when the prolonged services time threshold was met. Which service is primary is determined by the provider.

For example, a patient was seen in an office setting, including prolonged services, and then admitted to observation care by the same provider. The primary service was the observation care. List these codes:
- Code for the office setting with a modifier 25
- Code for observation care setting
- Prolonged services code +99418 (prolonged services in observation setting), since the primary service was the observation care.

Transfer from Observation to Inpatient Care
in Same Facility

Patient transferred from observation to inpatient care during a single stay by same provider.
- Report only an inpatient/observation code.

(continued on next page)

MULTIPLE SETTINGS – SAME PROVIDER (continued)
Transfer from Hospital Bed to Nursing Facility Bed in Same Facility
Patient transferred from a hospital bed to a nursing facility bed within the same facility by same provider. The facility has specific nursing facility beds. • This is considered to be two separate services because the patient was discharged from hospital care and admitted to a nursing facility bed. • Report two codes: a code for the discharge service; and a code for the initial nursing service.
Transfer from One Level of Care to Another Level in Same Facility
Patient transferred from one level of care to another level of care within a single facility (such as from a routine hospital unit to a critical care unit) by same provider. • This is not considered a new stay nor a transfer to a different facility. • Report only one code, not an initial care and another E/M service. For example, for an inpatient service and a critical care service in the same facility, report only the critical care code.
Discharge Services Followed by Other Services in Different Facility
Patient discharged from one facility and transferred to another facility by same provider. • This is considered a different stay. Report a subsequent care code for the second setting. • If code selection is based on time, report each service separately. The time for each service is counted separately. • Do **NOT** count the time spent on discharge services toward total time of the services in the other facility.   Do **NOT** count the time related to hospital inpatient or observation care in the initial facility (including admission and discharge services) to select a code for the subsequent service for other facility.
Discharge Services Followed by Other Services in Same Facility
Patient discharged from a facility and readmitted to same facility on the same date by same provider. • This is considered a single stay. • Report a subsequent care code, **NOT** a discharge or initial service code.
Consultation Services in One Location; Patient then Admitted to Hospital/Observation Care
Consultation provided in another location; same provider then admits the patient to initial inpatient/observation services care on the same date. Report two codes: a consultation code; and a subsequent hospital inpatient or observation care code.

(continued on next page)

MULTIPLE SETTINGS – DIFFERENT PROVIDERS
Consultation Services with Hospital/Observation Care **Different Providers**
Provider A performs a consultation service in anticipation of, or related to, the patient's admission by Provider B. Provider A then performs another consultation after the patient's admission. Provider A's second consultation is reported using a subsequent hospital inpatient/observation care code.
OTHER SERVICES
Do **NOT** report these codes with: • Admission services for a neonate (28 days of age or younger) requiring intensive observation, frequent interventions, and other intensive care services. Use 99477 instead. • Discharge services provided to newborns admitted and discharged on the same date. Use code 99463 instead. Do **NOT** report hospital discharge codes 99238, 99239 with • Initial hospital/observation care codes 99221, 99222, or 99223.

See next page for decision tree to help in selection of these codes.

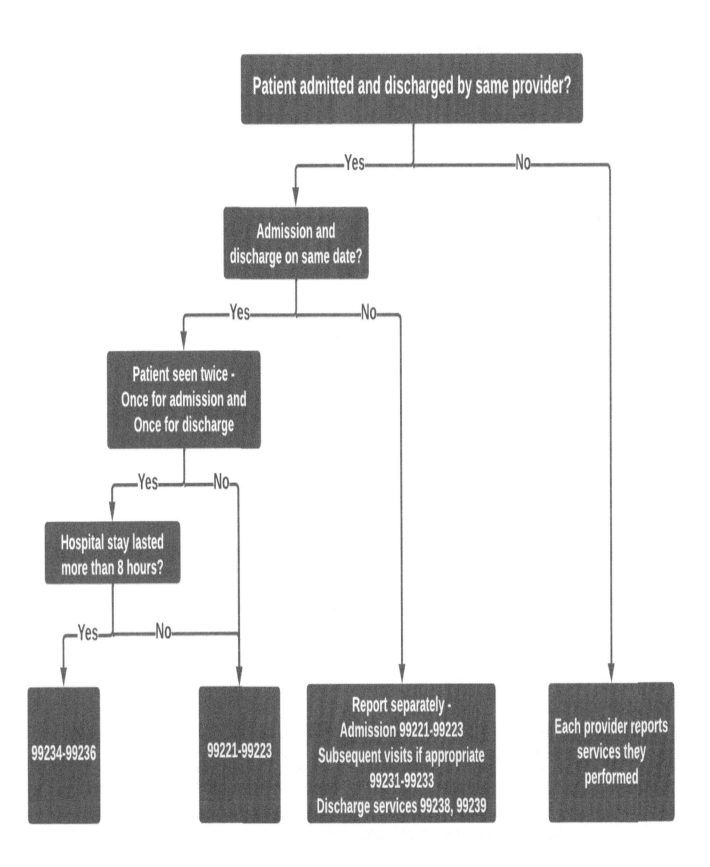

1. Which of these hospital/observation care codes do NOT include medical decision making?
   a. 99222
   b. 99234
   c. 99236
   d. 99238

2. An initial service is reported for hospital/observation care codes is defined as:
   a. When the patient has not received any previous professional services from the provider during this stay
   b. When the patient has not received any professional services from the provider during the last 3 years
   c. When the patient is being discharged from inpatient/observation care

3. A discharge code is reported when the patient was admitted on:
   a. On the same date
   b. On a different date

4. The provider saw the patient for 2 hours in the morning and 3 hours in the afternoon on the same day The time component is:
   a. 2 hours
   b. 3 hours
   c. 5 hours
   d. Reported with two separate codes, one for 2 hours in the morning and another for 3 hours in the afternoon.

5. The provider saw the patient at 11 pm on Tuesday and stayed with the patient until 2 am the next day. The time component is:
   a. 1 hour
   b. 2 hours
   c. 3 hours
   d. Reported with two separate codes, one for 11-12 pm and another for 12-2 am.

6. The coder is reporting a code for the second day that the patient is in observation care. The coder selected a code for:
   a. Initial service
   b. Subsequent service
   c. Discharge service
   d. Prolonged service

7. Provider performed a consultation in their office. Following the consultation, this same provider admitted the patient to the hospital. In this case, the coder selected:
   a. A code of the outpatient consultation and a code for the an initial inpatient code.
   b. A code for the outpatient consultation and a code for a subsequent inpatient service.
   c. Only a code for the outpatient consultation.
   d. Only a code for the initial hospital admission.

8. Dr. Smith performed a consultation in the emergency department. The patient was then admitted by Dr. Jones. After the admission, Dr. Smith saw the patient again in consultation. For Dr. Smith, the coder selected:
    a. A code for the consultation and another code for initial hospital care.
    b. A code for the consultation and another code for subsequent hospital care.
    c. A code for the consultation only.
    d. A code for the initial hospital care only.

9. Provider admits patient to the hospital at 9:00 am on Tuesday. The patient is hen discharged by the same provider at 3:00 on the same date. This is reported using:
    a. Same day admission and discharge codes
    b. Initial service codes
    c. Discharge service codes
    d. Initial and discharge service codes

See Appendix B for quiz answers.

Chapter 4

CPT® Consultations

A consultation is an E/M service provided at the request of another physician, other qualified health care professional, or appropriate source. The requesting provider asks the consultant to recommend care for a patient's specific condition or problem. Two providers must be involved.

See Appendix A for a form to assist in selecting an E/M code for these services.

Summary of Specific Criteria Used to Select Consultation Codes

Services	Correct Code Determined by -		
	Medically appropriate history and/or examination	MDM	Time
99242-99245 Office/Outpatient Consultations	√	√	√
99252-99255 Inpatient Consultations	√	√	√

To report an online or telephone consultation, see codes 99446-99452.

Specific Times and MDM Levels Used for Consultation Codes

Codes	Code selected using EITHER time measured in minutes or medical decision making	
	Time spent on date of service	Level of medical decision making
Office or Other Outpatient Consultations		
99242	20 minutes	Straightforward
99243	30 minutes	Low
99244	40 minutes	Moderate
99245	55 minutes	High
Inpatient or Observation Consultations		
99252	35 minutes	Straightforward
99253	45 minutes	Low
99254	60 minutes	Moderate
99255	80 minutes	High

Guidelines – All Consultation Services

GENERAL GUIDELINES
In a consultation, one provider asks another provider to recommend care for a patient's specific condition or problem.
These codes are reported by the consultant, **NOT** the requesting provider.
The consultant's opinion and any services that were ordered or performed must be communicated to the requesting provider by written report.
These services are provided either face-to-face with patient or using telemedicine services if appropriate.
There are no separate codes for new and established patients or initial and subsequent services.
There are separate codes for outpatient and inpatient consultations.
If a consultation is mandated (eg, required by a third-party payer), modifier 32 should added to the consultation code.

PROVIDERS
Only one consultation may be reported by a consultant per patient admission/encounter.
The consultant may initiate diagnostic and/or therapeutic services during the visit.
Consultations may be performed by: • Physician or other qualified health care professional.   • Appropriate source (non-clinical social worker, educator, lawyer, or insurance company).   • An advanced practice nurse or physician assistant working with the provider. They are considered as working in the exact same specialty and subspecialty as the provider. Only one or the other may report a consultation code for this patient during this encounter.
Do **NOT** report a consultation code if the encounter was initiated by the patient and/or family.

MULTIPLE SETTINGS
Consultation and Admission to Nursing Facility   **Same Provider**
Patient may be seen first for a consultation and then admitted to a nursing facility by the same provider on the same date. Report a code for the consultation and then a subsequent nursing facility code (99307-99310).

On the next pages are descriptions of outpatient consultation services and inpatient consultation services.

OUTPATIENT Consultation Services

Guidelines - OUTPATIENT Consultation Services (99242-99245)

GENERAL GUIDELINES
These codes are used for patients in these settings: • Office or other outpatient site. • Home or residence. • Emergency department. These services are provided either face-to-face with patient or using telemedicine services if appropriate. There are no separate codes for new and established patients or initial and subsequent services.
SELECTING CODES USING TIME OR MDM
These codes are selected using medical decision making or time. Sometimes the encounter lasts 15 minutes or longer than the time listed in in the highest level within a code category. If reporting the service by time, use prolonged services code +99417. Code +99417 can be listed in multiple units when appropriate. For example: • An office consultation lasted a total of 70 minutes. List code 99245 (55 minutes) plus +99217 (additional 15 minutes). • See Chapter 10 for more information on prolonged services.
ENCOUNTERS
Subsequent Consultations
There are no codes for subsequent consultations. • For subsequent outpatient consultations by the same provider, use an established patient code (99212-99215). • For a subsequent consultation in the patient's home, use a home or residence code (99347-99350). Subsequent consultations may be initiated by either the consultant or the patient.
MULTIPLE SETTINGS/SERVICES
Consultant Assumes Care for Patient
Patient seen for consultation. Primary provider then transfers patient's care to the same consultant. The consultant assumes management of either the patient's entire care or only the care of a specific condition or problem. Report two codes: a code for the consultation; and a code for the outpatient visit or home or residence services.
Outpatient Consultation and Hospital Inpatient/Observation Services **Same Provider**
Patient seen for consultation in outpatient setting, then admitted to inpatient/observation care by same provider on same date. Report two codes: one code for the outpatient consultation service; and a subsequent hospital inpatient or observation care code.

(continued on next page)

MULTIPLE SETTINGS/SERVICES (continued)
Consultation and Admission to Nursing Facility **Same Provider**
Patient may be seen first for an outpatient consultation and then admitted to a nursing facility by the same provider on the same date. Report two codes: a code for the consultation; and a subsequent nursing facility code (99307-99310).
Outpatient Consultation and Hospital Inpatient/Observation Services **Different Provider**
Patient seen for consultation on either the same date as the admission or on a prior date. For example: Provider A performs an outpatient consultation service in anticipation of, or related to, an admission by Provider B. Provider B then admits patient. Provider A then provides an inpatient consultation. Provider A reports two codes: an outpatient consultation code; and a subsequent hospital inpatient/observation care code. Provider B reports one code: the appropriate inpatient/observation care code.

INPATIENT Consultation Services

Guidelines - INPATIENT Consultation Services (99252-99255)

GENERAL GUIDELINES
These codes are used for patients in these settings: • Patients formally admitted as inpatients.   • Observation-level patients.   • Nursing facilities.   • Partial hospital setting.   These services are provided either face-to-face with patient or using telemedicine services if appropriate.   There are no separate codes for new and established patients or initial and subsequent services.
SELECTING CODES USING TIME OR MDM
Codes are selected using either medical decision making and time.   Time is reported by minute per day.   Sometimes the encounter lasts 15 minutes or longer than the time listed in the highest level within a code category. If reporting the service by time, use prolonged services code +99418. Code +99418 can be listed in multiple units when appropriate. For example: • An office consultation lasted a total of 95 minutes. List code 99255 (80 minutes) plus +99218 (additional 15 minutes).   • See Chapter 10 for more information on prolonged services.
PROVIDERS
A consultation service is reported when the provider or another provider from the same group practice has **NOT** provided any face-to-face service to this patient during this admission.   An advanced practice nurse or physician assistant may work with the provider. They are considered as working in the exact same specialty and subspecialty as the provider. Only one or the other may report a consultation service.
ENCOUNTERS
Subsequent Consultations
There are no codes for subsequent consultations. Patient was inpatient and then: • Another consultation by the same provider was performed in a home or residence setting. Use appropriate established patient code (99347-99350).   • Another consultation by the same provider was performed in the inpatient setting (same admission), Use appropriate subsequent care codes (99231-99233).   Subsequent consultations may be initiated by either the consultant or patient.
MULTIPLE SETTINGS/SERVICES
Consultant Assumes Care for Patient
Patient seen for inpatient consultation. Primary provider then transfers patient's care to same consultant. The consultant assumes management of either the patient's entire care or only the care of a specific condition or problem.   If care is then managed in an inpatient or observation setting, use appropriate code from inpatient/observation services code.   Report two codes: one for the consultation; and one for subsequent inpatient/ observation care.

(continued on next page)

MULTIPLE SETTINGS/SERVICES (continued)
Outpatient Consultation and Hospital Inpatient/Observation Services **Same Provider**
Patient seen for consultation in outpatient setting, then admitted to inpatient/observation care by same provider on same date. Report two codes: one code for the inpatient consultation service; and a subsequent hospital inpatient or observation care code.
Consultation and Admission to Nursing Facility **Same Provider**
Patient seen for an inpatient/observation care consultation and then admitted to a nursing facility by the same provider on the same date. Report two codes: • A code for the consultation and • A subsequent nursing facility code (99307-99310).
Outpatient Consultation and Hospital Inpatient/Observation Services **Different Provider**
Patient seen for consultation in outpatient setting then admitted to inpatient/observation care by a different provider on the same date of a prior date. For example: Provider A performs an outpatient consultation service in anticipation of, or related to, an admission by Provider B. Provider A then provides an inpatient consultation. Provider A reports two codes: an outpatient consultation code for the first visit; and a subsequent hospital inpatient/observation care code. Provider B reports one code; the appropriate inpatient/observation care code.

REVIEW – CHAPTER 4

1. Dr. Smith sees a patient in consultation in the hospital at the request of Dr. Jones. He renders an opinion. He then sends a report to Dr. Jones. What code should Dr. Smith use:
    a. Inpatient consultation code
    b. Initial inpatient hospital care code
    c. Subsequent hospital care code

2. A consultation can be provided:
    a. Only to inpatients
    b. Only to outpatients
    c. To either an inpatient or outpatient
    d. Only in the emergency room

3. A consultation may be provided by a:
    a. Physician
    b. Other qualified healthcare professional
    c. Non-clinical social worker
    d. Educator
    e. All of these professionals may report consultation codes

4. Dr. Lewis sees a patient in consultation in the hospital at the request of Dr. Ames. He renders an opinion. He then takes over the management of a portion of the patient's care. What code should Dr. Ames use to bill for his subsequent visits in his office:
    a. Inpatient consultation code
    b. Initial inpatient hospital care code
    c. Subsequent hospital care code
    d. Office/outpatient code (established patient)
    e. Office/outpatient code (new patient)

5. A mother asks for a consultation to discuss her child. The encounter takes place in the physician's office. This is reported as:
    a. Outpatient consultation
    b. Office or other outpatient service

6. This patient was seen in the provider's office for a consultation, then admitted by this provider to inpatient/observation care. This is reported using:
    a. Consultation code only
    b. Initial inpatient code only
    c. Both a code for the consultation and a code for initial inpatient care.
    d. Both a code for the consultation and a code for subsequent inpatient care.

See Appendix B for quiz answers.

Chapter 5

CPT® Emergency Services

An emergency department is defined as an organized hospital-based facility to provide unscheduled episodic services to patients who present for immediate medical attention. The facility must be available 24 hours a day.

Codes 99281-99285 are used to report evaluation and management services provided in the emergency department.

Code 99288 is used to report E/M services provided for emergency medical systems (EMS) emergency care, advanced life support, and patients being transported from one facility to another. This code does not include medical appropriate history and/or examination, medical decision making, or time.

Summary of Specific Criteria Used to Select Emergency Services Codes

Services		Correct Code Determined by -		
		Medically appropriate history and/or examination	MDM	Time
99281-99285	Emergency department services	√	√	
99288	Other emergency services			

These codes are **NOT** reporting using time because emergency department services typically vary greatly in the intensity of services required for patients and often involve multiple encounters with several patients over an extended period of time.

MDM Levels Used for Emergency Services

Codes	Code selected using medical decision making only
	Level of medical decision making
99281	None specified*
99282	Straightforward
99283	Low
99284	Moderate
99285	High
99288	None specified*

*Code 99281 does not require the presence of a physician or QHP. No MDM or time component is used with this code.

Code 99288 is used when a provider is communicating with emergency services personnel during patient transport. This code is also discussed in chapter 6.

The following pages discuss:

* Face-to-face emergency services
* Non-face-to-face emergency transport services

Guidelines - Emergency Services
FACE-TO-FACE (99281-99285)

GENERAL GUIDELINES

Services are provided in an organized hospital-based facility:
- Available 24 hours a day.
- For unscheduled episodic services.
- To patients who present for immediate medical attention.

These services are provided face-to-face with patient.

For a consultation in this setting, use outpatient consultation codes (99242-99245).

There are no separate codes for new and established patients or initial and subsequent services.

SELECTING CODES USING TIME OR MDM

These codes are selected using medical decision making only.

PROVIDERS

Codes 99282-99285 are reported for services provided by principal physician(s) and other qualified health care professional(s) who are overseeing the patient's care in a facility.

Code 99281 is reported for emergency department visits for patients that may **NOT** require the presence of a physician or other qualified health care professional.

An advanced practice nurse or physician assistant may work with the provider. They are considered as working in the exact same specialty and subspecialty as the provider. Only one or the other may report an emergency service.

MULTIPLE SETTINGS/SERVICES

Emergency Care Services in Observation or Inpatient Setting

Emergency-level services may be provided to a patient in observation status or inpatient setting.
- Report initial, subsequent or discharge inpatient or observation codes instead of emergency department codes.

Critical Care Services in Emergency Department

Critical care services may be provided in an emergency department setting. Report critical care codes only.

Emergency services for a patient were completed; patient then received critical care services. Report two codes: a code for the emergency services; and a code for the critical care services.

Emergency Services and other E/M services

Emergency services and another E/M services may be provided in different settings (such as hospital inpatient and observation care) or different facilities by same provider or group practice.

Coding depends on the circumstances:

- If only the other E/M services is being reported (not the emergency services), add together the total time spent in both settings.
- If emergency department codes are being reported, list two codes: a code for the emergency department services with a modifier 25; and a code for the initial admission to inpatient/observation care.

(continued on next page)

OTHER SERVICES
Services **NOT** included in these codes. Report separately if appropriate: • Procedures or other services identified by a CPT code. Add the appropriate modifier(s) to the other procedure/services. See chapter 18. • Emergency services that are related to a surgical package. Add the appropriate modifier(s) to the other procedure/services.
Do **NOT** report these codes: • For critical care services provided in the emergency department. Use codes 99291, +99292 instead. If the patient is seen in the emergency department for the convenience of the provider, use office or other outpatient services codes instead.

Guidelines - Emergency Medical Systems (EMS) Services
NON-FACE-TO-FACE (99288)

GENERAL GUIDELINES
This code is reported for provider's direction of emergency medical systems (EMS) for emergency care and advanced life support. The patient is being transported from one setting to another. Services include but are not limited to: • Telemetry of cardiac rhythm • Cardiac and/or pulmonary resuscitation • Endotracheal or esophageal obturator airway intubation • Administration of intravenous fluids • Administration of intramuscular, intratracheal or subcutaneous drugs • Electrical conversion of arrhythmia These services are provided non-face-to-face with patient (provider is not in the transport vehicle). There are no separate codes for new and established patients or initial and subsequent services.
SELECTING CODES USING TIME OR MDM
These codes are **NOT** reported using either medical decision making or time.
PROVIDERS
These services are provided by a physician or other qualified health care professional. Two entities are involved: • A provider located in a hospital emergency or critical care department and • Ambulance or rescue personnel located outside the hospital, in two-way voice communication with the provider.

1. Which one of these emergency services codes does NOT include medical decision making?
   a. 99282
   b. 99283
   c. 99284
   d. 99285
   e. 99288

2. Critical care and emergency-level services provided in observation area are reported using:
   a. Only the emergency department code
   b. Only the observation care code
   c. Both the emergency department code and the observation care code

3. Critical care and emergency department services were provided to a patient on the same date. The emergency services were completed; the patient's condition worsened and critical care services were provided. In this case:
   a. Report only the emergency department code
   b. Report only the critical care code
   c. Report both the emergency department code and the critical care code

4. For emergency medical systems services (99288), the provider (the individual reporting the code) is located:
   a. In a hospital emergency department or critical care department
   b. In an ambulance

5. A patient calls her physician about an acute condition. The physician asks her to meet him in the emergency room of a nearby hospital since it is halfway between the patient's home and the physician's office. This is reported using:
   a. An emergency department code
   b. An office/outpatient code
   c. A consultation code

6. Emergency services were provided to this patient. The patient was then admitted to observation care by the same provider. This is reported using:
   a. An emergency room code only. Add together the time spent in each setting to select the appropriate code.
   b. An observation code only. Add together the time spent in each setting to select the appropriate code.

See Appendix B for quiz answers.

Chapter 6

CPT® Critical Care Services

Critical care services are provided by a physician or other qualified health care professional to patients who have a critical illness or injury. Critical care typically but not always requires interpretation of multiple physiologic parameters and/or application of advanced technology(s).

Summary of Specific Criteria Used to Select Critical Care Codes

Code	Age of Patient	Services	Time
Codes Used in a Variety of Settings			
99291	Varies	Face-to-face services Outpatient care – Any age Inpatient care – Age over 5 years old Critical care transport – Age over 24 months	First 30-74 minutes
+99292	Varies	Face-to-face services Outpatient care – Any age Inpatient care – Age over 5 years old Critical care transport – Age over 24 months	Each additional 30 minutes
Codes Used for Patient During Transport			
99288	Over 24 months	Non-face-to-face services	No time specified
99466	24 months or younger	Face-to-face services Provider with patient during transport	First 30-74 minutes
+99467	24 months or younger	Face-to-face services Provider with patient during transport	Each additional 30 minutes
99485	24 months or younger	Non-face-to-face services Provider directing services during transport	First 30 minutes
+99486	24 months or younger	Non-face-to-face services Provider directing services during transport	Each additional 30 minutes
Inpatient Critical Care			
99468	28 days or younger	Face-to-face services Initial inpatient service	Per day
99469	28 days or younger	Face-to-face services Subsequent inpatient service	Per day
99471	29 days through 24 months	Face-to-face services Initial inpatient service	Per day
99472	29 days through 24 months	Face-to-face services Subsequent inpatient service	Per day
99475	2 years through 5 years	Face-to-face services Initial inpatient service	Per day
99476	2 years through 5 years	Face-to-face services Subsequent inpatient service	Per day

Many of the services for the different types of critical care overlap. However, there are some differences in specific services, wording used to describe these services and specific codes listed for the services. These are described on the next page.

Comparison of the Services Included in
the Different Critical Care Codes

Services included in pediatric/neonate transport codes (provider physically in transport vehicle): 99466, +99467*	Services included in critical care codes: 99291, +99292	Services included in inpatient neonatal/ pediatric critical care codes: 99468, 99469, 99471, 99472, 99475, 99476**
Blood gases and information data stored in computers (eg, ECGs, blood pressures, hematologic data)	Blood gases – collection and interpretation of physiological data (eg, ECGs, blood pressures, hematologic data)	Monitoring and interpretation of blood gases or oxygen saturation (94760-94762)
Gastric intubation (43752, 43753)	Gastric intubation (43752, 43753)	Oral or nasogastric tube placement (43752)
Vascular access procedures (36000, 36400, 36405, 36406, 36415, 36591, 36600)	Vascular access procedures (36000, 36410, 36415, 36591, 36600)	Vascular access procedures (36000, 36140, 36400, 36405, 36406, 36420, 36510, 36555, 36600, 36620, 36660)
Ventilatory management (94002, 94003, 94660, 94662)	Ventilatory management (94002-94004, 94660, 94662)	Airway and ventilation management (31500, 94002-94004, 94375, 94610, 94660)
Pulse oximetry (94760-94762)	Pulse oximetry (94760-94762)	Pulse oximetry (94760-94762)
Cardiac output measurements (93598)	Cardiac output measurements (93598)	Cardiac output measurements (93598)
Chest x-rays (71045, 71046)	Chest x-rays (71045,71046)	Chest x-rays (71045,71046)
Temporary transcutaneous pacing (92953)	Temporary transcutaneous pacing (92953)	Temporary transcutaneous pacing (92953)
Routine monitoring evaluations (eg, heart rate, respiratory rate, blood pressure, pulse oximetry)		Transfusion of blood components (36430, 36440)
		Suprapubic bladder aspiration (51100)
		Bladder catheterization (51701, 51702)
		Lumbar puncture (62270)
		Car seat evaluation (94780-94781)

*Services included in transport codes 99485, +99486, 99288 (provider is **NOT** in the transport vehicle) include providing treatment advice to transport team and reviewing data submitted by the transport team.

**The services in the right hand column are also included in neonatal/infant intensive care services.

Services on these lists may **NOT** be reported separately by providers, but **MAY** be reported separately by facilities.

Services **NOT** on these lists may be reported separately.

GENERAL GUIDELINES

Provider assesses, manipulates, and supports vital system function(s) to treat single or multiple vital organ system failure(s) and/or prevent further life threatening deterioration of condition.

Vital organ system failure may include: central nervous system failure, circulatory failure, shock, renal, hepatic, metabolic, and/or respiratory failure.

These codes all include high complexity MDM.

Codes are determined by:
- Location of the services (inpatient, outpatient or patient in transport),
- Whether the services are face-to-face with patient or non-face-face (transport services)
- Age of the patient (neonatal, pediatric patients and older patients)

There are no separate codes for new and established patients.

Services may be provided on multiple days, even if there is no change in the patient's condition.

SELECTING CODES USING TIME And/or MDM

These codes are selected using time and medical decision making. MDM is always high.

PATIENTS

Patient's condition/injury:
- Acutely impairs one or more vital organ systems.
- Has a high probability of imminent or life-threatening deterioration in patient's condition.

Do **NOT** report these codes if patient is:
- Not critically ill but happens to be in critical care area
- Not critically ill but requires intensive observation, frequent interventions, and other intensive care services. Use intensive care services code 99477-99480 instead.

PROVIDERS

Do **NOT** report these codes if provider is:
- Performing services to another patient during the same period of time.

OTHER SERVICES

See chart on previous page for a list of included services. These services may be reported separately by facilities, but not by providers.

Services **NOT** included in these codes. Report separately if appropriate:
- Other E/M services on same day by same provider.

The following pages describe the different types of critical care services:
- Critical care provided in OUTPATIENT setting
- Critical care provided in INPATIENT setting
- Critical care provided during PATIENT TRANSPORT from one facility to another (face-to-face with patient and non-face-to-face).

Note that codes 99291 and +99292 are listed in all the different categories (outpatient, inpatient and patient transport) but with different criteria in each category.

Critical Care Services in OUTPATIENT Settings

Summary of Outpatient Critical Care Services

Codes		Correct Code Determined by -			
		Medically appropriate history and/or examination	MDM	Time	Age
99291	Outpatient critical care		High	First 30-74 minutes	Any age
+99292	Outpatient critical care		High	Each additional 30 minutes	Any age

See chart in CPT book that describes times for coding for 99291 and add-on code +99292.

Guidelines - Critical Care Services in OUTPATIENT Settings (99291, +99292)

GENERAL GUIDELINES

Use these codes for outpatient critical care for services (any age) in an office/other outpatient settings, including:
- Physician's office
- Hospital clinic
- Emergency room

Codes may be reported over multiple days if patient's condition continues to be critical. This applies even if no changes are made in the treatment being given.

These services are provided face-to-face with patient.

There are no separate codes for new and established patients or initial and subsequent services.

SELECTING CODES USING TIME AND/OR MDM

These codes are selected using time and medical decision making (high only).

Time may or may not be continuous.

Time must be recorded in patient's medical record.

Time must be spent providing direct care to an individual patient.

These services are reported by minutes:
- Report 99291 once per date for first 30-74 minutes.
- Report +99292 for each additional 30 minutes. This code may be reported in multiple units when appropriate.

Sometimes a patient is unable to participate in discussions related to their care. In this case, discussions may include family members or surrogate decision makers on floor or unit.
Time spent in these discussions may be included in calculating critical care time. The discussion must be directly related to management of the patient. These discussions may include time spent:
- Obtaining medical history.
- Reviewing patient's condition or prognosis.
- Discussing treatment or limitations of treatment.

Do **NOT** report these codes:
- If total time is less than 30 minutes.
- If provider spends any time providing services to another patient during this service time.

(continued on next page)

GUIDELINES – CRITICAL CARE SERVICES (99291, +99292)
MULTIPLE SETTINGS/SERVICES
Multiple Services provided by Same Provider or Group Practice
Critical care provided in both outpatient and inpatient care settings on same date by same physician: • Use critical care codes (99468-99472) for all services on that date.
Care provided in emergency department completed; patient's condition worsens, requiring inpatient critical care: • Use both emergency department and critical care codes.
Patient in intensive care, then becomes critically ill. Patient referred to another physician in same group practice: • Physician reports initial critical care codes only.
MULTIPLE PROVIDERS
Patient received critical care services from two providers during the same time period. Second individual is: • Of different specialty than other provider AND • Not reporting per day neonatal or pediatric critical care Each provider can report critical care codes for their services.
OTHER SERVICES
Providers may **NOT** report these codes, but facilities **MAY** do so: • Blood gases – collection and interpretation of physiological data (eg, ECGs, blood pressures, hematologic data) • Gastric intubation (43752, 43753) • Vascular access procedures (36000, 36410, 36415, 36591, 36600) • Ventilatory management (94002-94004, 94660, 94662) • Pulse oximetry (94760-94762) • Cardiac output measurements (93598) • Chest x-rays (71045,71046) • Temporary transcutaneous pacing (92953)
Services **NOT** included in these codes. Report separately if appropriate: • Codes for other E/M services provided on the same day by same provider. • Other services or procedures. Do **NOT** include time to provide these other services in calculating critical care time.
Do **NOT** report these codes: • With other services provided on the same date, by the same individual or by a different individual of same specialty or same group.

Critical Care Services in INPATIENT Settings

Inpatient critical care codes are defined by medical decision making (high level only), time and age of patient.

Summary of Inpatient Critical Care Services

Codes		Correct Code Determined by -			
		Medically appropriate history and/or examination	MDM	Time	Age
99468	Inpatient critical care		High	Initial service Per day	28 days or younger
99469	Inpatient critical care		High	Subsequent service Per day	28 days or younger
99471	Inpatient critical care		High	Initial service Per day	29 days through 24 months
99472	Inpatient critical care		High	Subsequent service Per day	29 days through 24 months
99475	Inpatient critical care		High	Initial service Per day	2 years through 5 years
99476	Inpatient critical care		High	Subsequent service Per day	2 years through 5 years
99291	Inpatient critical care		High	First 30-74 minutes	Age over 5 years old
+99292	Inpatient critical care		High	Each additional 30 minutes	Age over 5 years old

Guidelines - Critical Care Services in INPATIENT Settings
(99468, 99469, 99471, 99472, 99475, 99476, 99291, +99292)

GENERAL GUIDELINES

Inpatient critical care services are usually provided in a critical care area, such as coronary care unit, intensive care unit, pediatric intensive care unit, respiratory care unit or emergency care facility.

Codes are selected according to age of the patient:
- Use codes 99468, 99469 for patients 28 days or younger.
- Use codes 99471, 99472 for patients 29 days through 24 months.
- Use codes 99475, 99476 for patients 2 through 5 years of age.
- Use codes 99291, +99292 for patients older than 5 years.

These services are provided either face-to-face with patient or non-face-to-face (eg, on floor or unit).

There are no separate codes for new and established patients.

There are separate codes for initial and subsequent services.

SELECTING CODES USING TIME AND/OR MDM

These codes are selected using medical decision making (high only) and time.

Total time may not be continuous.

Time must be recorded in patient's medical record.

Time must be spent providing direct care to an individual patient, either at bedside or on unit/floor.

Include minutes spent at patient's bedside or on floor or unit. Time may be spent:
- Reviewing test results or imaging studies.
- Discussing patient care with other medical staff.
- Documenting services in the medical record.

Codes 99291, +99292 are reported by specific minutes spent with patient per day.
- Report 99291 once per date for first 30-74 minutes.
- Report +99292 for each additional 30 minutes. This code may be reported in multiple units when appropriate.

Codes 99468, 99469, 99471, 99472, 99475, 99476 are reported for services per day, according to age of patient. No specific times are included.

ENCOUNTERS

Use initial care codes (99291, 99468, 99471, 99475) once per hospital admission.

MULTIPLE SETTINGS/TYPES OF SERVICES

Patient Received Both Outpatient and Inpatient Care On Same Date
Same Provider

On same date, patient received both outpatient and inpatient care by same physician:
- Use critical care codes (99468-99472) for all services on that date.

Patient Received Emergency Care and Critical Care
Same Provider

Patient's emergency department care completed. Patient's condition worsens; then requires critical care:
- Use both emergency department and critical care codes.

(continued on next page)

MULTIPLE SETTINGS/TYPES OF SERVICES (continued)
Patient Received Critical Care Services and Hospital Care or Intensive Services **Same Provider**
Patient received both critical care services and hospital care or intensive care services from one physician or group. • Use only code for critical care services (99468, 99471, 99475).
Patient Received Normal Newborn Service, Then Required Critical Care **Same Provider**
Patient received normal newborn services (99460-99462); then became critically ill. Use two codes: • Code 99468 for initial critical care with modifier 25 and • Code for newborn service.
Patient aged 28 days or younger is discharged from critical care; then readmitted to critical care. • Use code 99469 for first day of readmission and any additional days of critical care.
Patient aged 29 days through 24 months is discharged from critical care; then readmitted to critical care. • Use code 99472 for first day of readmission and any additional days of critical care.
Patient Received Critical Care in Outpatient and Inpatient Settings **Same Provider**
Patient younger than 6 years old received care in both outpatient and inpatient settings. • Use critical care codes (99468-99476) for all services.
MULTIPLE PROVIDERS
Patient received critical care services from two providers during the same time period. Second individual may use code 99291, +99292 if provider is: • Of different specialty than other provider AND • Not reporting per day neonatal or pediatric critical care. NOTE: If both providers are in same specialty, only one provider can report critical care codes.
Patient in Intensive Care; Referred for Critical Care on Same Date **Different Providers/Different Group Practice**
Patient in intensive care; then becomes critically ill. Patient referred to another provider (receiving provider) on same date. • <u>Referring</u> provider reports only one code, such as time based intensive care codes, hospital care services, or normal newborn services. • <u>Receiving</u> individual reports pediatric or neonatal critical care codes (99468-99476).
Patient Transferred to Another Provider during Same Hospital Stay **in Same Facility**
During same hospital stay in same facility: • Provider A (transferring physician) provides critical care services and then transfers patient to • Provider B (receiving physician) who provides a lower level of care such as intensive or subsequent hospital care. <u>Transferring</u> provider - Use subsequent hospital/observation care codes or critical care codes 99291, +99292. <u>Receiving</u> provider – Use codes for lower level of service as appropriate. If patient then readmitted to critical care with Provider A, this provider uses codes for subsequent critical care codes (99469, 99472, 99476).

(continued on next page)

MULTIPLE PROVIDERS (continued)
Patient Transferred to Another Provider in a Different Facility
On same day, care provided to patients younger than 6 years at two separate facilities by physicians of different groups. • <u>Referring provider</u> transfers patient from their facility. Use codes 99291, +99292 based on time for services provided in their facility. • <u>Receiving provider</u> in another facility on the same date. Use codes 99468, 99471, 99475 for services provided in their facility.
OTHER SERVICES
Providers may **NOT** report these services separately, but facilities **MAY** do so. • Monitoring and interpretation of blood gases or oxygen saturation (94760-94762) • Oral or nasogastric tube placement (43752) • Vascular access procedures (36000, 36140, 36400, 36405, 36406, 36420, 36510, 36555, 36600, 36620, 36660) • Airway and ventilation management (31500, 94002-94004, 94375, 94610, 94660) • Pulse oximetry (94760-94762) • Cardiac output measurements (93598) • Chest x-rays (71045,71046) • Temporary transcutaneous pacing (92953) • Transfusion of blood components (36430, 36440) • Suprapubic bladder aspiration (51100) • Bladder catheterization (51701, 51702) • Lumbar puncture (62270) • Car seat evaluation (94780-94781)
Do **NOT** use 99291, +99292 with codes 99468-99476 for services by same provider or different individual of same specialty in same group on same date.

85

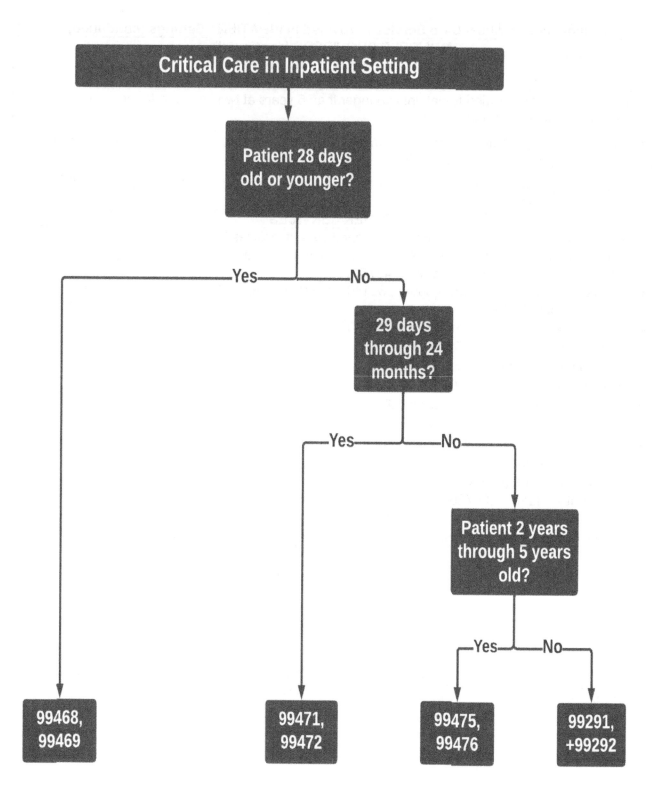

Critical Care in Inpatient Setting

Patient 28 days old or younger?

Yes — No

29 days through 24 months?

Yes — No

Patient 2 years through 5 years old?

Yes — No

99468, 99469

99471, 99472

99475, 99476

99291, +99292

Critical Care During Patient Transport

Critical care patient transport codes (patient being transported from one facility to another) care codes are defined by medical decision making, time and age of patient.

There are separate codes for when provider is in the vehicle with the patient and for when the provider is **NOT** in the vehicle with the patient.

Critical Care During Patient Transport From One Facility to Another Facility
(Provider PHYSICALLY PRESENT In Transport Vehicle)

Summary of Face-to-Face Patient TRANSPORT Services

Codes		Correct Code Determined by -			
		Medically appropriate history and/or examination	MDM	Time	Age
99466	Critical care transport		High	First 30-74 minutes	24 months or younger
+99467	Critical care transport		High	Each additional 30 minutes	24 months or younger
99291	Critical care transport		High	First 30-74 minutes	Over 24 months
+99292	Critical care transport		High	Each additional 30 minutes	Over 24 months

Critical Care During Patient TRANSPORT From One Facility to Another

These guidelines apply to:
- Services provided <u>face-to-face</u> with patient
- Services provided by <u>physician or other qualified healthcare professional who is physically in the transport vehicle</u> with the patient

Patient Transport Services (Codes 99291, +99292, 99466, +99467)

GENERAL GUIDELINES
Use codes 99466, +99467 for patients 24 months or younger.
Use codes 99291, +99292 for patients over 24 months.
There are no separate codes for new and established patients or initial and subsequent services.

SELECTING CODES USING TIME OR MDM
Codes are selected using time and medical decision making (high only).
Time: • <u>Begins</u> when physician assumes primary responsibility for a patient at the referring facility   • <u>Ends</u> when receiving facility accepts responsibility for the patient's care   • Includes only time spent face-to-face with patient during transport.
Do **NOT** use these codes: • If time is less than 30 minutes face-to-face with patient. Use other appropriate E/M code.
• Report code 99291 once per date, initial 30-74 minutes for patients over 24 months.   • Report +99292 for each additional 30 minutes for patients over 24 months. This code may be reported in multiple units when appropriate.
• Report code 99466 once per date, initial 30-74 minutes for patients 24 months or younger.   • Report code +99467 for each additional 30 minutes per date for patients 24 months or younger. This code may be reported in multiple units when appropriate.

PATIENTS
The patient is in critical condition and therefore requires care during the transfer.

PROVIDERS
Provider is physically in the transport vehicle with the patient.

OTHER SERVICES
Providers may **NOT** report these services separately, but facilities **MAY** do so: • Blood gases and information data stored in computers (eg, ECGs, blood pressures, hematologic data)   • Gastric intubation (43752, 43753)   • Vascular access procedures (36000, 36400, 36405, 36406, 36415, 36591, 36600)   • Ventilatory management (94002, 94003, 94660, 94662)   • Pulse oximetry (94760-94762)   • Cardiac output measurements (93598)   • Chest x-rays (71045, 71046)   • Temporary transcutaneous pacing (92953)   • Routine monitoring evaluations (eg, heart and respiratory rate, blood pressure, pulse 0ximetry)

(continued on next page)

88

OTHER SERVICES (continued)

Services **NOT** included in these codes. List separately if appropriate:
- Pre-transport communication between control (directing) physician and referring facility before or following patient transport
- Critical care provided in referring facility prior to transfer (99291, +99292)
- Total body and selective head cooling of neonates (99184).
- For services provided:
  - <u>After</u> patient arrived at receiving facility. Report other codes (hospital-based services).
  - <u>Before</u> patient transported (still in referring facility). Report critical care codes 99291, +99292.

Do **NOT** report separately:
- Procedures or services performed by other members of transporting team.
- With non-face-to-face critical care transport services (99485, +99486) for same patient, by same physician on the same date.

Critical Care During Patient TRANSPORT From One Facility to Another Facility (Non-face-to-face)

These guidelines apply to:
- Services provided <u>non-face-to-face</u> with patient
- Services provided by <u>physician or other qualified healthcare professional who is **NOT** physically in the transport vehicle</u> with the patient

For transport service when the provider is in the transport vehicle with the patient, see page 88.

Summary of Non-Face-to-Face Patient TRANSPORT Services

Codes		Correct Code Determined by -		
		Medically appropriate history and/or examination	Time	Age
99485	Critical care transport		First 30 minutes	24 months or younger
+99486	Critical care transport		Each additional 30 minutes	24 months or younger
99288*	Critical care transport, advanced life support		No time specified	Over 24 months

*Code 99288 is also discussed in Chapter 5.

GENERAL GUIDELINES

Services reported for all two-way communication between control (directing) physician and specialized transport team and reviewing data collected:
- Prior to transport.
- At the referring facility.
- During transport of patient back to receiving facility.

Code 99288 includes but is not limited to the services listed below. Services performed by the transport team under direction of the provider may include:
- Direction of telemetry of cardiac rhythm
- Cardiac and/or pulmonary resuscitation
- Endotracheal or esophageal obturator airway intubation
- Administration of intravenous fluids
- Administration of drugs (Intramuscular, intratracheal or subcutaneous)
- Electrical conversion of arrhythmia.

There are no separate codes for new and established patients or initial and subsequent services.

SELECTING CODES USING TIME OR MDM

Codes are selected using time only. Total time may not be continuous.

Time spent with transport team and reviewing data must be recorded.

Time:
- Begins with first contact with specialized transport team.
- Ends when patient's care is handed over to team at receiving facility.

Do **NOT** use these codes:
- If total time is 15 minutes or less. Use another E/M code.

- Use code 99485 once on a given date for first 16-45 minutes.
- Use code +99486 for each additional 30 minutes per date. This code may be reported in multiple units when appropriate.
- Code 99288 does not include a specific time.

PATIENTS

These services are provided to a patient being transported from one facility to another.

The patient is in critical condition and therefore requires care during the transport.

Use codes 99485, +99486 for patients 24 months or younger.

Use code 99288 for patients older than 24 months.

(continued on next page)

Guidelines - Services During Patient TRANSPORT (Codes 99485, +99486, 99288)
(Provider NOT in vehicle) (continued)

PROVIDERS

Provider is **NOT** physically in the transport vehicle with the patient.

Two entities are involved:
- A control/directing provider located in a hospital emergency or critical care department and
- Ambulance or rescue personnel located outside the hospital, in two-way voice communication with the provider.

These codes are reported by the control (directing) provider.

Control (directing) physician:
- Provides treatment advice to transport team who are with patient and providing hands-on care.
- Reviews data submitted by transport team

Services may be provided both in original facility and other facility where patient is being transferred:
- Referring provider transfers patient from their facility. Use codes 99291, +99292 based on time for services provided in their facility.
- Receiving provider in another facility on the same date. Use codes 99468, 99471, 99475 for services provided in their facility.

OTHER SERVICES

Services **NOT** included in these codes. List separately if appropriate:
- Pre-transport communication between controlling (directing) physician and referring facility before or after patient transport.
- Critical care provided in referring facility prior to transfer (99291, +99292).
- Services provided after patient has been admitted to receiving facility, such as:
  - Emergency department services (99281-99285).
  - Initial hospital care (99221-99223).
  - Critical care (99291, +99292).
  - Initial neonatal intensive care (99477).
  - Critical care (99468).

Do **NOT** report these codes:
- With face-to-face critical care transport codes (99466, +99467) for same patient, same physician on the same date.
- For procedures or services provided by members of transporting team.

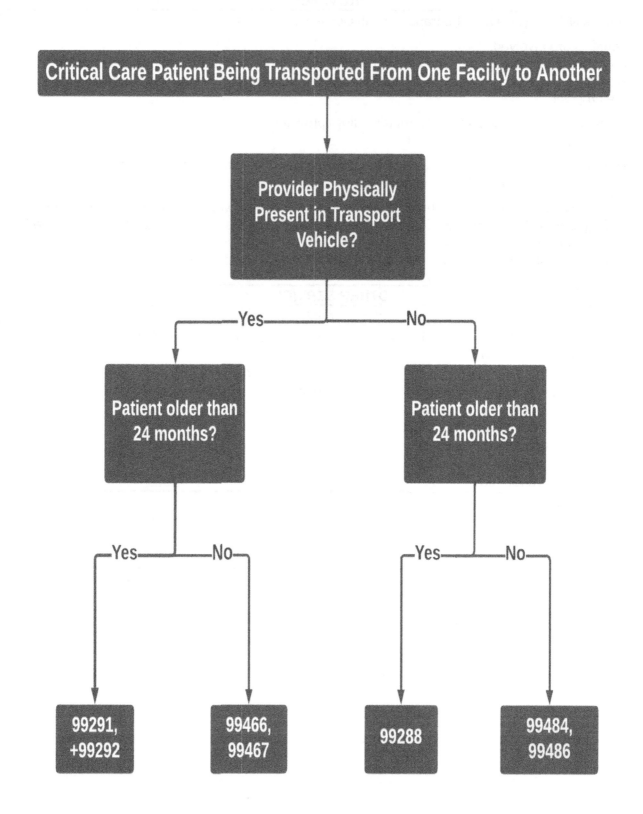

Critical Care Patient Being Transported From One Facilty to Another

Provider Physically Present in Transport Vehicle?

- Yes
  - Patient older than 24 months?
    - Yes → 99291, +99292
    - No → 99466, 99467
- No
  - Patient older than 24 months?
    - Yes → 99288
    - No → 99484, 99486

1. This patient received critical care services in the Emergency Department. The time providing these services is documented as 2-1/2 hours. The coder should:
   a. List a code from the Emergency Department
   b. List codes 99291 and +99292x3.
   b. List codes +99292x3 only.
   d. List code 99291x3

2. Which of these critical care codes is NOT selected using minutes spent with patient:
   a. 99291
   b. 99466
   c. 99476

3. Which of these critical care codes are reported for non-face-to face services:
   a. 99466
   b. +99467
   c. 99485
   d. +99468

4. A critically ill patient, under age 24 months, is being transported from one facility to another, with provider in the vehicle with the patient. These services are reported using:
   a. 99466
   b. 99291
   c. +99292
   d. 99486

5. Vascular access procedures are included in:
   a. Pediatric/neonate transport codes
   b. Critical care codes
   c. Inpatient neonatal and pediatric care codes
   d. All of these services

6. A patient is located in a critical care area but is not currently critically ill. In this case:
   a. Report a critical care code
   b. Report other appropriate code

7. Codes 99291 and +99292 can be reported for services provided for:
   a. Outpatient care, patient up to 71 months
   b. Critical care transport, patient over 24 months
   c. Inpatient care, patient 6 years or older
   d. These codes can be used In all these circumstances

8. For reporting face-to-face time for critical care pediatric and newborn transport codes (99466, +99467), begin counting time when:
   a. The physician assumes primary responsibility for a patient at the referring facility
   b. When the facility accepts responsibility for the patient from the patient
   c. When the physician enters the transport vehicle
   d. When the patient enters the transport vehicle

9. For reporting non-face-to-face time for critical care pediatric and newborn transport codes (99485, +99486), begin counting time when:
    a. The physician enters the transport vehicle
    b. The patient enters the transport vehicle
    c. The provider has first contact with specialized transport team (in the transporting vehicle)
    d. The patient's care is handed over to the receiving facility

10. A critically ill pediatric patient is transferred from one facility to another on the same date. The <u>receiving</u> physician at the new facility reports:
    a. Codes 99468, 99471 or 99475 as appropriate
    b. Codes 99291, +99292

11. Two providers are performing critical care services during the same time period. The providers are of different specialties and neither are reporting per day critical care services. In this case:
    a. Only one provider can report critical care codes
    b. Neither provider can report critical care codes
    c. Each provider reports their own critical care codes

12. Codes 99291, +99292 can be used in any of these settings EXCEPT:
    a. Outpatient settings
    b. Inpatient settings
    c. Patient transport; provider is in vehicle with patient
    d. Patient transport; provider is not in vehicle with patient

See Appendix B for quiz answers.

Chapter 7

CPT® Neonatal and Pediatric Intensive Care Services

Intensive care services are provided to neonates and pediatric patients who are not critically ill but require intensive observation, frequent interventions, and other intensive care services. This is considered a lower level of care than critical care. Codes are selected by codes by weight of baby at time of birth and weight of baby at time of the encounter.

Summary of Criteria Used to Select Neonatal Intensive Care Codes

Code	Initial or Subsequent Hospital Care	Patient
99477	Initial	Neonate – 28 days of age or younger No body weight specified
99478	Subsequent	Very low weight infant Present body weight less than 1500 grams
99479	Subsequent	Recovering low birth weight infant Present body weight of 1500-2500 grams
99480	Subsequent	Recovering low birth weight infant Present body weight 2501-5000 grams

Guidelines – Neonatal Intensive Care Services (99477-99480)

GENERAL GUIDELINES

Services provided to pediatric patients who are not critically ill but require intensive observation, frequent interventions, and other intensive care services.

Codes are selected using:
- Age of neonate (older than 28 days or younger than 28 days).
- Birth weight (low or very low) and current weight of child (except code 99477).

These services are provided face-to-face with patient.

There are separate codes for initial or subsequent service.

There are no separate codes for new and established patients

SELECTING CODES USING TIME OR MDM

Codes are reported once per day for each provider and each patient in a facility.

No specific number of minutes per day are indicated.

PATIENTS

These codes are used for an infant with a diagnosis of low or very low birth weight:
- Low weight at birth, current weight 1500-2500 grams (99479)
- Very low weight at birth, current weight less than 1500 grams (99478)
- Recovering from low birth weight, current weight 2500-500 grams (99480)
- Neonate requiring intensive care services but no weight mentioned – neonate 28 days of age or younger (99477)

(continued on next page)

PROVIDERS
• Health care team under direct supervision of physician or other qualified health care professional. • Only one individual may report these codes.

MULTIPLE PROVIDERS/SETTINGS
Multiple Providers During Same Hospital Stay – Patient Transferred In and Out of Intensive Care
Patient seen by multiple providers during same hospital stay; transferred in and out of intensive care during same hospital stay (but not same date). For example: • Provider A performs intensive care services. • Patient then discharged to lower level of service to receive care from Provider B. • Patient then readmitted to receive intensive care from Provider A. • Provider A reports two codes: code 99479 for first day of intensive care and then codes 99478-99480 for days after readmission.
Transferring/Receiving Providers – Patient Transferred From Intensive Care to Lower Level of Care
Both services provided <u>on same date</u>: • <u>Transferring individual</u> provided initial intensive care to patient, then transferred the patient to a lower level of care on same date. Reports neonate intensive care (99477). • <u>Receiving individual</u> provided a lower level of care. Reports either subsequent hospital care (99231-99233) or subsequent normal newborn care (99460-99462) as appropriate.
Both services provided <u>on different dates</u>: • <u>Transferring individual</u> provided initial intensive care to patient, then transferred the patient to a lower level of care. Reports subsequent hospital care (99231-99233) for this date. (May have provided intensive care services on initial date). • <u>Receiving individual</u> provided a lower level of care. Reports either subsequent hospital care (99231-99233) or subsequent normal newborn care (99462) as appropriate.
Transferring/Receiving Providers – Patient Transferred From Intensive Care to Critical Care
Neonate or infant received intensive care; then becomes critically ill and is transferred to critical care unit.
Services provided from individual from <u>different groups</u>: • <u>Transferring individual</u> provided either initial or subsequent intensive care and then transfers the patient to critical care. Reports EITHER critical care services (99291, +99292) for time spent providing this care or initial or subsequent intensive care (99477-99480) but not both. • <u>Receiving individual</u> provides critical care. Reports initial or subsequent critical care service (99468-99476).
Services provided by <u>same provider or providers from same group practice</u>: • Report only initial or subsequent critical care (99468-99476).

(continued on next page)

OTHER SERVICES

Services **NOT** included in these codes. Report separately if appropriate:
- Other procedures performed as a <u>necessary</u> part of resuscitation such as endotracheal intubation (31500) performed as part of pre-admission delivery room care. If performed as a convenience (not necessary) prior to patient's admission to neonatal intensive care unit, do **NOT** report separately.
- Attendance at delivery with initial intensive care services (99464). List two codes: 99464 and intensive care code 99477 with modifier 25.
- Delivery/birthing room resuscitation with initial intensive care services (99465). List two codes: 99465 and intensive care service code 99477 with modifier 25.

Providers may **NOT** report these services separately, but facilities **MAY** do so.
- Monitoring and interpretation of blood gases or oxygen saturation.
- Oral or nasogastric tube placement (43752).
- Vascular access procedures (36000, 36140, 36510, 36555, 36400, 36405, 36406, 36420, 36600, 36620, 36660).
- Airway and ventilation management (31500, 94002-94004, 94375, 94610, 94660).
- Pulse oximetry (94760-94762).
- Cardiac output measurements (93598).
- Chest x-rays (71045, 71046).
- Temporary transcutaneous pacing (92953).
- Transfusion of blood components (36430, 36440).
- Suprapubic bladder aspirations (51100).
- Bladder catheterization (51701, 51702).
- Lumbar puncture (62270).
- Car seat evaluation (94780, 94781).
- Intensive cardiac and respiratory monitoring.
- Continuous and/or frequent vital sign monitoring.
- Heat maintenance.
- Enteral and/or parenteral nutritional adjustments.
- Laboratory and oxygen monitoring.
- Constant observation by the health care team under direct supervision of the physician or other qualified health care professional.

Do **NOT** use these intensive care codes:
- For ill neonate not requiring intensive care. Use 99221-99223 instead.
- For inpatient care of normal newborn. Use 99460 instead.
- For subsequent care of sick neonate younger than 28 days of age but more than 500 grams when neonate does not require intensive or critical care services. Use 99231-99233 instead.
- For initiation of services for critically ill neonate. Use 99468 instead.

1. Some neonatal services overlap with services associated with critical care codes. A service included in both neonatal and critical care codes is:
   a. Heat maintenance
   b. Oral or nasogastric tube placement
   c. Laboratory and oxygen monitoring
   d. Enteral and/or parenteral nutritional adjustments

2. Sometimes a patient will receive both intensive care and critical care on the same date from providers who are in the same group practice. In this case, report:
   a. Critical care code only
   b. A critical care code and an intensive care code
   c. Intensive care code only

3. Dr. A provides intensive care. By the next day, the patient no longer needs intensive care, although the baby is still ill. Dr A transfers the infant to Dr. B within the same facility (but not the same group) to provide critical care services. Dr. B reports:
   a. Initial or subsequent critical care
   b. Subsequent intensive care
   c. Subsequent hospital care
   d. Initial hospital care

4. Most neonatal and pediatric intensive care codes are reported by current body weight. The exception is:
   a. 99477
   b. 99478
   c. +99489
   d. 99480

5. A patient may receive intensive care on one day, then be discharged to a lower level of service, but then readmitted to intensive care. For the day of readmission to intensive care, use codes:
   a. Initial intensive care 99477
   b. Subsequent intensive care 99478-99480
   c. Initial hospital inpatient services 99231-99333

6. Which of these elements in NOT part of neonatal and pediatric intensive care services:
   a. Patient is critically ill
   b. Patient requires intensive observation
   c. Patient requires frequent interventions

See Appendix B for quiz answers.

Chapter 8

CPT® Nursing Facility Services

Nursing facility services codes are used to report services in: a nursing facility; a skilled nursing facility; a psychiatric residential center; or in an intermediate care facility for individual with intellectual disabilities.

The place of service (POS) code on the claim form will indicate the specific type of service being reported. The POS codes are listed in the front of the CPT book. For these services, the codes are:
- Nursing facilities - 32
- Skilled nursing facilities - 31
- Psychiatric residential treatment center - 56
- Intermediate care facility for individuals with intellectual disabilities - 54

Federal and state regulations pertaining to the care of nursing facility residents determine:
- The nature and minimum frequency of assessments and visits.
- Who may perform the initial comprehensive visit.

For care plan oversight for a patient in a nursing facility, see codes 99379, 99380. These are discussed in chapter 12.

See Appendix A for a form to assist in selecting an E/M code for these services.

Summary of Criteria Used to Select Nursing Facility Services

Codes	Correct Code Determined by -		
	Medically appropriate history and/or examination	MDM	Time
99304-99310 Nursing facility services	√	√	√
99315-99316 Nursing facility discharge services			√

Specific Times and MDM Levels Used for Nursing Facility Codes

Codes	Most codes selected using EITHER time measured in minutes or medical decision making	
	Time spent on date of service	Level of medical decision making
Initial Nursing Facility Care		
99304	25 minutes	Straightforward or Low
99305	35 minutes	Moderate
99306	50 minutes	High
Subsequent Nursing Facility Care		
99307	10 minutes	Straightforward
99308	20 minutes	Low
99309	30 minutes	Moderate
99310	45 minutes	High
Nursing Facility Discharge Services		
99315	30 minutes	
99316	More than 30 minutes	

Guidelines – Nursing Facility Services (99304-99310, 99315, 99316)

GENERAL GUIDELINES
These codes are used to report evaluation and management services to patients in: • Nursing facilities • Skilled nursing facilities • Psychiatric residential treatment center • Intermediate care facility for individuals with intellectual disabilities. For a consultation in this setting, use inpatient consultation codes 99252-99255. There are separate codes for initial or subsequent service. There are no separate codes for new and established patients. See section on next page on special guidelines for MDM for these services.

(continued on next page)

SELECTING CODES USING TIME OR MDM
Time

Codes 99304-99310 are reported either by total minutes per day or medical decision making.

Codes 99315-99316 are reported by minutes only.

If multiple visits occur over the course of a single calendar date in the same setting, a single service is reported.
- If the code is being selected using MDM, use the aggregated MDM over the course of the calendar date. See the guidelines below for information about a component of MDM used only for these codes.

- If the code is being selected using time, sum the time over the course of the day using the guidelines for reporting time.

The encounter may last 15 minutes or longer than the time listed in the highest level within a code category (initial service [50 minutes] or subsequent service [45 minutes]). If time is being used to select the level of service, use prolonged services code +99418. Code +99418 can be listed in multiple units when appropriate.
- For example, a subsequent patient encounter lasted a total of 60 minutes. List two codes: 99310 (45 minutes) and +99218 (additional 15 minutes).
- See Chapter 10 for more information on prolonged services.

Medical Decision Making (MDM)

MDM for nursing facility codes include an additional category within the element of Number and Complexity of Problems Addressed at the Encounter. This is used only for codes requiring a high-level MDM (99306, 99310).

This new category is: Multiple morbidities requiring intensive management. This is defined as a set of conditions, syndromes, or functional impairments that:
- Are likely to require frequent medication changes or other treatment changes and/or re-evaluations.
- Place the patient at a significant risk of worsening medical (including behavioral) status and risk for (re)admission to a hospital.

For the other categories of MDM, the elements (amount and/or complexity of data to be reviewed and analyzed and the risk of complications and/or morbidity or mortality of patient management) are the same as for other services.

(continued on next page)

CPT© codes and descriptions only copyright 2023 American Medical Association. All right reserved.
Other content copyright Medical Coding Made Easy LLC © 2023 All Rights Reserved.

PROVIDERS
The provider who oversees the care of the patient in the facility is referred to as the principal provider or admitting physician. • The principal provider may work with others but oversees the overall medical care of the patient, in order to provide timely care to the patient. • Other providers may be specialists who perform consultations or concurrent care. An advanced practice nurse or physician assistant may work with the provider. They are considered as working in the exact same specialty and subspecialty as the principal provider and therefore cannot report services as specialists, consultants or providers of concurrent care. Modifiers may be required to identify the role of the individual performing the service. See chapter 18.
MULTIPLE SETTINGS
Transfer From a Skilled Nursing Facility to a Nursing Facility Level of Care Same Facility Same Provider
Patient is transferred from a skilled nursing facility to a nursing facility level of care. This is considered the same stay. Report only one code: an initial service code.
Transfer From Another Site to a Nursing Facility Setting Same Provider
Patient was seen in another site (eg, hospital emergency department, office) and then admitted to a nursing facility during the same encounter. Report two codes: a code for initial site with a modifier 25, and a code for nursing facility admission.
Patient was seen in another site and then admitted to nursing facility care as a consultation by same provider on the same date. Report two codes: one for the initial site and one for a subsequent nursing facility care.
Discharge from Hospital/Observation Care; Admitted or Readmitted to Nursing Facility
Patient discharged from hospital or observation care on the same date and then admitted or readmitted to a nursing facility. Report two codes: one for the discharge services and one for the nursing facility admission.

(continued on next page)

CPT© codes and descriptions only copyright 2023 American Medical Association. All right reserved.
Other content copyright Medical Coding Made Easy LLC © 2023 All Rights Reserved.

ENCOUNTERS

Initial Encounter

Initial services are provided face-to-face with patient.

Federal and state regulations pertaining to the care of nursing facility residents determine:
- The nature and minimum frequency of assessments and visits.
- Who may perform the initial comprehensive visit.

CPT guidelines state:

Initial service for <u>skilled nursing facility</u> care must be provided by a physician.

Initial service for <u>nursing facility</u> care may be provided by physician or other qualified health care professionals, if allowed by state law or regulation.

Use initial services codes:
- Only once per admission, per physician or QHP, regardless of length of stay.
- When the patient has not received any face-to-face professional services from a physician or QHP of the exact same specialty and subspecialty who belongs to the same group practice. An advanced practice nurse or physician assistant is considered to be in the exact same group and subspecialty as the physician.
- The patient is a new patient as defined in the E/M guidelines (eg, three year requirement).

Subsequent Encounters

Subsequent services are provided face-to-face or using telemedicine services if appropriate.

Discharge Services (99315-99316)

Codes are selected based only on the total time of the discharge management provided in a face-to-face encounter.

The face-to-face encounter with the patient and/or family/caregiver may be performed on a date prior to the date the patient actually leaves the facility.

Time spent with the patient may or may not be continuous.

The discharge codes include, as appropriate:
- Final examination of the patient.
- Discussion of the nursing facility stay.
- Instructions for continuing care given to all relevant caregivers.
- Preparation of discharge records, prescriptions, and referral forms.

OTHER SERVICES

Do **NOT** report:
- Initial services codes 99304-99306 more than once per admission, per provider.

1. For E/M coding, a psychiatric residential treatment facility is considered:
   a. An observation care unit
   b. A rest home
   c. Emergency room care
   d. a nursing facility

2. This patient has been in a nursing facility for 6 months. She is now being released to her home. The coder should select a code for:
   a. Initial service
   b. Subsequent service
   c. Discharge service
   d. Prolonged service

3. Nursing facility services include a new element in medical decision making. This new element, multiple morbidities requiring intensive management, is used only in this category of MDM:
   a. Number and complexity of problems addressed
   b. Amount and/or complexity of data to be reviewed
   c. Risk of complication and/or morbidity or mortality of patient management

4. For initial skilled nursing care, the service must be provided by:
   a. Physician
   b. Clinical staff
   c. Other qualified healthcare professional
   d. Advance care nurse

5. A patient was first seen in the hospital emergency room and then admitted to nursing facility. In this case:
   a. Report both the emergency room and nursing facility codes
   b. Report only the emergency department code
   c. Report only the nursing facility code

6. A patient was seen for a consultation in the physician's office and then admitted to a nursing facility. In this case:
   a. Report both the outpatient consultation and an initial nursing facility code
   b. Report both the outpatient consultation and a subsequent nursing facility code
   c. Report only the outpatient consultation code
   d. Report only the initial nursing facility code

7. All of these services are reported with nursing facilities codes EXCEPT:
   a. Care plan oversight
   b. Skilled nursing facilities
   c. Intermediate care facility for individuals with intellectual disabilities
   d. Psychiatric residential treatment center

See Appendix B for quiz answers.

Chapter 9

CPT® Home or Residence Services

These codes are used to report E/M services provided in a home or residence setting.

See Appendix A for a form to assist in selecting an E/M code for these services.

For care plan oversight for a patient in home or residence setting, see codes 99374, 99375. These are discussed in chapter 12.

Summary of Criteria Used to Select Home or Residence Codes

Codes		Correct Code Determined by -		
		Medically appropriate history and/or examination	MDM	Time
99341, 99342, 99344, 99345	Home or residence services, New patient	√	√	√
99347-99350	Home or residence services, Established patient	√	√	√

Specific Times and MDM Levels Used for Home or Residence Codes

Codes	Most codes selected using EITHER time or medical decision making	
	Time spent on date of service	Level of medical decision making
New Patients		
99341	15 minutes	Straightforward
99342	30 minutes	Low
99344	60 minutes	Moderate
99345	75 minutes	High
Established Patients		
99347	20 minutes	Straightforward
99348	30 minutes	Low
99349	40 minutes	Moderate
99350	60 minutes	High

GENERAL GUIDELINES

Home is defined as a(n):
- Private residence
- Temporary lodging
- Short-term accommodation (eg, hotel, campground, hostel, or cruise ship)
- Assisted living facility
- Group home (not licensed as an intermediate care facility for individuals with intellectual disabilities)
- Custodial care facility
- Residential substance abuse treatment facility

These services are provided face-to-face with patient.

For a consultation in this setting, use outpatient consultation codes 99242-99245.

There are separate codes for new and established patients.

There are no separate codes for initial and subsequent services.

SELECTING CODES USING TIME OR MDM

These codes are selecting using either time or medical decision making.

Time is calculated by minutes.

The encounter may last 15 minutes or longer than the time listed in in the highest level in a code category (new patient [75 minutes] or established patient [60 minutes]). If time is being used to select the level of service, use prolonged services code +99417. Code +99417 can be listed in multiple units when appropriate.

- For example, a new patient encounter lasted a total of 90 minutes. List code 99345 (75 minutes) plus +99217 (additional 15 minutes).

- See Chapter 10 for more information on prolonged services.

Do **NOT** count time spent travelling to or from patient's home or residence.

ENCOUNTERS

These codes can be reported for a follow-up consultation in the patient's home.

OTHER SERVICES

Do **NOT** report the following services using home or residence codes:

- An initial consultation provided to a patient in a home or residence. Use an office or other outpatient consultation code instead.

- Oversight services provided in a domiciliary, rest home (eg, assisted living facility), or home setting. Use care management services codes +99437, 99491, or principal care management codes 99424, +99425 instead.

- Services provided to patients with intellectual disabilities in intermediate care facility setting. Use nursing facility codes instead.

- Services provided in a psychiatric residential treatment center setting. Use nursing facility services codes instead.

- A patient admitted to either hospital inpatient/observation status, or to a nursing facility in the course of an encounter in another setting. Use initial hospital inpatient/ observation care or initial nursing facility care codes instead.

1. Home or residence codes are NOT used for services provided in:
   a. Private residence
   b. Group home
   c. Residential substance abuse facility
   d. Intermediate care facility for individuals with intellectual disabilities

2. A patient is seen in his home for an initial consultation. In this case:
   a. Report an outpatient consultation code
   b. Report an inpatient consultation code
   c. Report an outpatient consultation code and a home or residence code

3. If selecting a home or residence code using time, count:
   a. Time spent with patient and time spent going to and from the patient's home
   b. Time spent with patient only
   c. Time is not part of these codes

See Appendix B for quiz answers.

Chapter 10

CPT® Prolonged Services

Prolonged services codes are used with a primary E/M code when the time listed in the primary code is exceeded (time spent with patient is more than the time listed in the code).

Codes are selected by:
- The location of the service
- The provider of the service (physician, QHP or clinical staff)
- Whether or not the services were on the same date as a face-to-face E/M service.

Most of these are add-on codes used only with other E/M codes. The except is code 99358.

Most codes are added to the highest level of service in a category. The exceptions are 99358, +99359.

Most codes are added to a primary E/M code selected by time only. The exception is +99415, 99358

Summary of Criteria Used to Select Prolonged Services Codes

Codes		Correct Code Determined by -			
		Setting	Direct Contact (face-to-face) with patient?	Same day as face-to-face with patient?	Time
+99415	Prolonged clinical staff services	Outpatient	Yes	-	First hour
+99416	Prolonged clinical staff services	Outpatient	Yes	-	Each additional 30 minutes
+99417	Prolonged services on same date as other E/M services	Outpatient	Maybe	Yes	15 minutes
+99418	Prolonged services	Inpatient, observation or nursing facility	Maybe	Yes	15 minutes
99358	Prolonged services on date other than face-to-face service	Outpatient, inpatient or observation	No	No	First hour
+99359	Prolonged services on date other than face-to-face service	Outpatient, inpatient or observation	No	No	Each additional 30 minutes

The following pages include general guidelines that apply to all prolonged services codes and then specific guidelines for the different categories of these codes.

GENERAL GUIDELINES
These codes are added to a primary E/M code for a related service.
The related service may or may not be on the same date as the prolonged service. • Some prolonged codes can only be added to the highest level of code within a category, while others can be added to any code within a category. • Some prolonged codes can be added to a primary code selected using time only, while others can be added to a related code selected by either MDM or time.
Codes +99415-99417 are reported for encounters in office/outpatient settings.
Codes +99418 is reported for encounters in inpatient, observation or nursing facility settings.
Codes 99358, +99359 are reported for encounters in outpatient, inpatient or observation settings.
Services may be provided face-to-face with patient, using telemedicine services if appropriate, or non-face-to-face, depending on the specific code.
SELECTING CODES USING TIME OR MDM
These codes are reported using time only.
These codes may be added to codes for services provided on the same date or on a different date than the related services, depending on the specific code.
PROVIDERS
Services may be provided by clinical staff or physician or other qualified healthcare professional, depending on the specific code.

Each of these types of services are described beginning on the next page:
• Prolonged care provided in OUTPATIENT setting
• Prolonged care provided in INPATIENT setting
• Critical care provided in NURSING FACILITY setting.

At the end of this chapter are decision trees to help in selection of inpatient and outpatient prolonged services.

Prolonged Services in OUTPATIENT Settings

The guidelines on this page apply to:
- Prolonged services in <u>outpatient</u> settings
- Services that were <u>face-to-face</u> with patient and/or family/caregiver
- Services provided by <u>clinical staff</u>
- Services on <u>same date</u> as primary E/M service

Prolonged Services (Codes +99415, +99416)

GENERAL GUIDELINES
Codes +99415, +99416 are reported in addition to the primary outpatient E/M services code provided at the same session by clinical staff.
There are no separate codes for new and established patients or initial and subsequent services.
SELECTING CODES USING TIME OR MDM
Primary codes may be selected by time or medical decision making.
Prolonged services codes are selected using time only.
The prolonged service must exceed the time listed in the primary code by at least 30 minutes.
These codes are added to the highest level of primary code in the category (such as 99205 but not 99202-99204).
Time may not be continuous. In this case, use only the time spent by clinical staff face-to-face with patient or the family/caregiver.
Report +99415 for first hour of prolonged services on a given date.
Report +99416 for each additional 15 minutes of prolonged services on a given date. This code can be reported in multiple units as appropriate.
Code +99416 can also be used to report the final 15-30 minutes of prolonged service on a given date.
Do **NOT** count time spent in providing other services in calculating time for prolonged services.
Do **NOT** report: <ul><li>Code +99415 for prolonged services of less than 30 minutes total on a given date.</li><li>Code +99416 for prolonged services of less than 15 minutes beyond the first hour.</li><li>Code +99416 for less than 15 minutes beyond the final 30 minutes.</li></ul>
PROVIDERS
Report these codes for services provided face-to-face with patient by clinical staff.
Physician or other QHP is present to provide direct supervision of clinical staff.
Clinical staff may not report +99415, +99416 for more than two simultaneous patients. If treating two patients, the prolonged services time is calculated separately for each patient.
OTHER SERVICES
Do **NOT** report: <ul><li>Code +99416 with code +99417</li><li>Code +99415 or +99416 with code +99417</li></ul>
These codes can **NOT** be reported by facilities.

Prolonged Services in OUTPATIENT Settings (continued)

The guidelines on this page apply to:
- Prolonged services in <u>outpatient</u> settings
- Services provided <u>with or without face to face</u> contact with patient and/or family/caregiver
- Services provided by <u>physician or other qualified healthcare professional</u>
- Services on <u>same date</u> as primary E/M service

Prolonged Services (Code +99417)

GENERAL GUIDELINES
Code +99417 is reported in addition to the primary outpatient E/M services code provided at the same session by physician or other qualified healthcare professionals.
Services are provided face-to-face with patient and/or non-face-to-face or using telemedicine services if appropriate.
There are no separate codes for new and established patients or initial and subsequent services.

SELECTING CODES USING TIME OR MDM
Primary code was selected using time only.
Prolonged services code is selected using time only.
Cognitive assessment and care plan services code 99483 does not have a time threshold, only a typical time (60 minutes). If this typical time is exceeded by at least 15 minutes, use add-on code +99417.
These codes are added to the highest level of primary code in a category (such as 99205 but not 99202-99204).
The prolonged service must exceed the time listed in the primary code by at least 15 minutes.
Time spent with and without direct patient contact may be added together.
Report +99417 for each additional 15 minutes of prolonged services on a given date. This code can be reported in multiple units when appropriate.
Do **NOT** report code +99417 for prolonged services of less than 15 minutes total on a given date.
Do **NOT** count time spent performing separately reported services when calculating time for primary E/M code and prolonged services code.

PROVIDERS
Report these codes for services provided by physicians or other qualified healthcare professionals.

OTHER SERVICES
Use code +99417 with: • Outpatient service (99205, 99215) • Outpatient consultations (99245) • Home or residence visit (99345, 99350) • Cognitive assessment when typical time is exceeded by 15 minutes (99483)
Do **NOT** report +99417 on same date of services as: • Psychotherapy add-on codes (+90833-+90838) • Prolonged services on date other than face-to-face service (99358-+99359) • Prolonged clinical staff services (+99415, +99416)

Prolonged Services in INPATIENT AND OBSERVATION Settings

The guidelines on this page apply to:
- Prolonged services in <u>inpatient and observation</u> settings
- Services provided <u>with or without face to face contact</u> with patient and/or family/caregiver
- Services provided by <u>physician or other qualified healthcare professional</u>
- Services on <u>same date</u> as primary E/M service

Prolonged Services (Code +99418)

GENERAL GUIDELINES
Code +99418 is reported in addition to the primary inpatient/observation E/M services code provided at the same session by a physician or other qualified healthcare professional.
Services are provided face-to-face with patient, non-face-to-face or using telemedicine services if appropriate.
There are no separate codes for new and established patients or initial and subsequent services.

SELECTING CODES USING TIME OR MDM
Primary code was selected using time only. Services may be provided with face-to-face time with patient combined with non-face-to-face time.
These codes are added to the highest level of primary code in a category (such as 99255 but not 99252-99254).
The prolonged service must exceed the time listed in the primary code by at least 15 minutes.
Report +99418 for each additional 15 minutes of prolonged services on a given date. This code can be reported in multiple units when appropriate.
Do **NOT** report code +99418:
• For prolonged services of less than 15 minutes total on a given date.
Do **NOT** count time spent performing separately reported services when calculating time for primary E/M code and prolonged services.

PROVIDERS
Report these codes for services provided by physicians or other qualified healthcare professionals.

OTHER SERVICES
Report code +99418 with highest level of service in a category. Use this code with: • Hospital inpatient/observation care (99223, 99233, 99236) • Inpatient consultations (99255) • Nursing facility care (99306, 99310)
Do **NOT** use +99418 on same date of services as: • Psychotherapy add-on codes (+90833, +90836, +90838) • Prolonged services on date other than face-to-face service (99358, +99359)

The guidelines on this page apply to:
- Prolonged services in <u>inpatient and observation</u> settings
- Services provided <u>non-face-to-face</u> with patient and/or family/caregiver
- Services provided by <u>physician or other qualified healthcare professional</u>
- Services on <u>different date</u> as primary E/M service

Prolonged Services (Codes 99358, +99359)

GENERAL GUIDELINES
The primary service is related to: • A face-to-face service with the patient that has or will occur on a different date than these services and • Ongoing patient management. An example of these service is extensive record review after or before the date a patient is seen. Code 99358 is **NOT** an add-on code. Code +99359 is an add-on code. Services provided non-face-to-face with patient by physician or qualified healthcare professional. There are no separate codes for new and established patients or initial and subsequent services.
SELECTING CODES USING TIME OR MDM
Primary codes was selected using time or medical decision making. Prolonged services codes are selected using time only. The prolonged service must exceed the time listed in the primary code by at least 30 minutes. These codes are added to any primary code if services provided on a different date. It is not necessary that the primary code be the highest level in a category. Time may not be continuous. Use code 99358 only once per date for first hour of prolonged services. Report +99359 for each additional 15 minutes of prolonged services. It can also be reported for final 15 to 30 minutes of prolonged service on a given date. This code can be reported in multiple units when appropriate. Do **NOT** report these codes if prolonged time is: • Less than 30 minutes beyond the primary code. Report primary code only. • Less than 15 minutes beyond the final 30 minutes.
PROVIDERS
Services provided by physician or other qualified healthcare professional.

(continued on next page)

Prolonged Services (Codes 99358, +99359)

OTHER SERVICES
Do **NOT** report 99358, +99359 on the same date as: • Office or other outpatient services (99202-99205, 99212-99215) • Hospital inpatient or outpatient care (99221-99223, 99231-99236) • Office or other outpatient consultations (99242, 99243, 99244, 99245) • Inpatient or observation consultations (99252-99255) • Emergency department services (99281-99285) • Nursing facility services (99304-99310) • Home or residence services (99341-99345, 99347-99350) • Other prolonged services codes (+99417, +99418) • Cognitive assessment and care plan services (99483) Do **NOT** report 99358, +99359 with these services if the other service does not include patient contact. For example: • Care plan oversight services (99374-99380) • Chronic care management (99347, 99491) • Principal care management (99424-99427) • Home and outpatient INR monitoring (93792, 93793) • Medical team conferences (99366-99368) • Interprofessional telephone/Internet/electronic health record consultations, or online digital evaluation and management services) (99446-99452) • Online digital E/M services (99422-99423).

A decision tree on the next page describes coding for prolonged services.

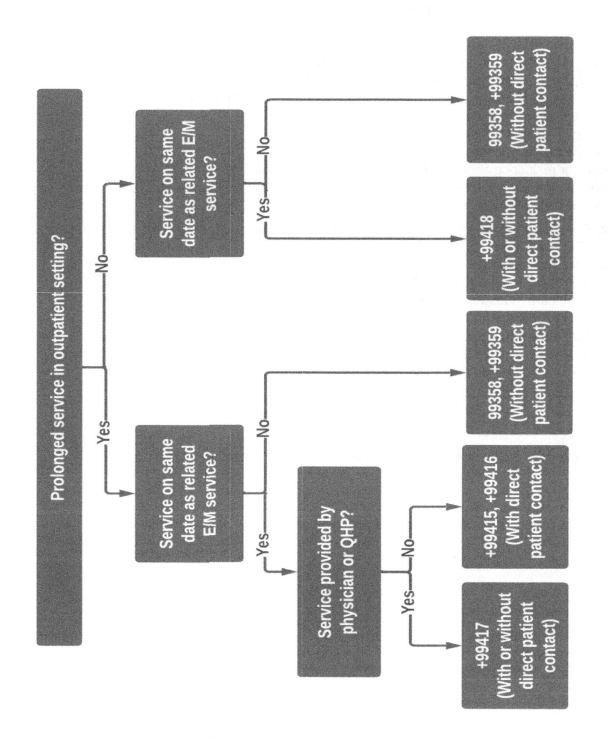

1. Prolonged services codes 99358 and +99359 can only be reported for services provided:
   a. On day of related face-to-face services with patient
   b. On day other than day of related face-to-face services with patient
   c. On either day of or day before or after the day of a related face-to-face service with patient

2. Prolonged services codes +99415 and +99416 can only be reported for services provided:
   a. In an office or outpatient setting
   b. In an inpatient or observation setting
   c. In either an office or inpatient/observation setting

3. Prolonged services codes +99418 and +99417 can only be reported for services provided:
   a. Face-to-face only
   b. Non-face-to-face only
   c. Either or both face-to-face and non-face-to-face

4. Sometimes an E/M service is provided, with prolonged services, and also other services such as a test or diagnostic procedure. In this case:
   a. Include the other services in counting the prolonged services time
   b. Do not include the other services in counting the prolonged services time

5. A new patient was seen in a face-to-face encounter with clinical staff in the office setting (99205) under the supervision of a physician. The encounter lasted 2 hours. In this case, report code:
   a. 99205, +99415, +99416
   b. 99205, +99415
   c. 99205, +99416

6. A provider reviewed test results the day following a face-to-face visit with a patient. The review time was for 80 minutes. In this case:
   a. 99358
   b. 99358 and +99359
   c. 99358 and +99359x2

See Appendix B for quiz answers.

118

Chapter 11

CPT® Preventive Medicine Services

Preventive medicine codes are reported for a patient who is not currently sick (does not have either a diagnosis or signs or symptoms of a condition). An example would be an annual check-up or a well-baby visit.

Some preventive services codes include different sets of codes for new and established patients and age of patient.

Some preventive services codes include time.

Summary of Criteria Used to Select Preventive Medicine Services

Codes		Different codes for New or Established patient?	Age	Time
99381-99387, 99391-99397	Preventive Medicine	Yes	√	
99401-99404	Preventive medicine, individual counseling	Yes		√
99406-99409	Behavior change Interventions, individual	No		√
99411-99412	Preventive medicine, group counseling	No		√

Note that these services differ as follows:
- The preventive medicine services codes (99381-99387, 99391-99397) include a comprehensive history and examination and age appropriate counseling. These are not further defined. No time is included.

- The counseling codes (99401-99404, 99411-99412) include counseling only. No history or examination is required. They do not list specific behaviors that are the focus of the encounter.

- The behavior change intervention codes (99406-99409) include counseling/intervention. No history or examination is required. Specific behaviors are the focus of the encounter (smoking, alcohol abuse, or substance abuse).

Each of these types of services are described on the next pages.

Preventive Medicine Services

These codes are used to report the preventive medicine E/M service for infants, children, adolescents, and adults.

The examination required for these codes is described as "comprehensive" but specific components required for the examination are not listed.

The extent and focus of the services will largely depend on the age of the patient. For example, the appropriate history, examination and counseling for a 14 year old girl would be very different that the appropriate history, examination and counseling for a 45 year old man.

Specific Ages Used to Select for Preventive Care Codes

Codes	Codes selected using Age of Patient
New Patients	
99381	Infant (younger than 1 year)
99382	Early childhood (1 through 4 years)
99383	Late childhood (5 through 11 years)
99384	Adolescence (12 through 17 years)
99385	18 through 39 years
99386	40 through 64 years
88387	65 years or older
Established Patients	
99391	Infant (younger than 1 year)
99392	Early childhood (1 through 4 years)
99393	Late childhood (5 through 11 years)
99394	Adolescence (12 through 17 years)
99395	18 through 39 years
99396	40 through 64 years
99397	65 years or older

Preventive Medicine Services (99381-99387, 99391-99397)

GENERAL GUIDELINES

The service includes:
- Age and gender appropriate history.
- Age and gender appropriate examination.
- Counseling/anticipatory guidance/risk factor reduction interventions.
- Ordering of laboratory/diagnostic procedures.

These services may be provided in a physician's office, hospital clinic, home, or rest home.

These services are provided face-to-face with patient.

There are separate codes for new and established patients.

There are no separate codes for initial and subsequent services.

SELECTING CODES USING TIME OR MDM

These codes are **NOT** selected using either time or medical decision making.

No MDM is needed since the patient is not sick or injured, and therefore the provider does not need to establish a diagnosis or select a management option (the requirements for MDM).

PATIENTS

Codes are selected by patient's age and whether or not the patient is new or established to the provider.

OTHER SERVICES

Laboratory/diagnostic procedures are often performed/ordered during preventive visits. Examples are:
- Vaccine/toxoid administration and products.
- Vaccine risk/benefit counseling.
- Ancillary studies involving laboratory, radiology, other procedures, or screening tests.

Ordering these procedures is included in preventive services. Do **NOT** report separately. Performing these procedures is **NOT** included. Report separately.

Other E/M services may be performed with these codes, depending on the nature of the problem involved. These may be problems:
- Discovered during the examination
- Mentioned by the patient during examination
- A pre-existing problem addressed during the encounter.

If the problem is considered significant,* report the E/M service separately with a modifier 25. If the problem is considered insignificant,* do **NOT** report a E/M service separately.

Do **NOT** report these codes if:
- Counseling was part of another E/M service being reported (such as 99401-99404, 99406-99409, 99411, 99412)

* A significant problem requires the physician to perform additional work, including the components of an E/M service (medical decision making and/or time) to assess the condition or symptom. Use the appropriate E/M code to report the additional work required. Report two codes: a preventive medicine service code; and another E/M service with modifier 25.

An insignificant or trivial problem does **NOT** require the physician to perform additional work. No additional E/M code is listed. List only a preventive medicine service code.

Preventive Medicine, Counseling and/or Risk Factor Reduction

These services are provided to a patient in order to promote the patient's health and prevent illness or injury.

Codes are selected by type of counseling (individual or group) and time spent with the patient.

Specific Times Used to Select for Counseling and/or Risk Factor Reduction Codes

Codes	Codes Selected Using Time Spent with Patient
Individual Counseling	
99401	Approximately 15 minutes
99402	Approximately 45 minutes
99403	Approximately 30 minutes
99404	Approximately 60 minutes
Group Counseling	
99411	Approximately 30 minutes
99412	Approximately 60 minutes

Preventive Medicine, Counseling and/or Risk Factor Reduction (99401-99404, 99411, 99412)

GENERAL GUIDELINES

Report these services for counseling for patients with conditions/concerns such as:
- Family problems
- Diet
- Exercise
- Substance use
- Sexual practices
- Injury prevention
- Dental health
- Diagnostic/laboratory test results.

No history or examination is required.

Use codes 99401- 99404 for <u>individual</u> counseling.

Use codes 99411, 99412 for <u>group</u> counseling.

These services are provided face-to-face with patient.

There are no separate codes for new and established patients or initial and subsequent services.

SELECTING CODES USING TIME OR MDM

Codes are selected using time only.

Do **NOT** use these codes to report time spent counseling when the same time is also part of any other E/M services that were provided at the same encounter.

(continued on next page)

PATIENTS
The patient does **NOT** have a specific illness for which counseling might be otherwise be provided.

PROVIDERS
Services provided by physician or other qualified healthcare provider.

OTHER SERVICES
Services **NOT** included with these codes. Report separately if appropriate: • Other distinct services on same day. Report separately with modifier 25
Do **NOT** report these codes: • With health behavior assessment and intervention services (96156, 96158, 96159, 96164-96168, 96170, 96171) if provided on same day. • When the patient is receiving counseling associated with a problem (diagnosis or symptom).

Behavior Change Interventions, Individual Counseling

These codes are reported for services provided to persons who exhibit a specific behavior that is often considered an illness in itself. These codes may be reported when performed:
- For treatment of conditions related to or potentially exacerbated by the behavior OR
- To change a harmful behavior that has not yet resulted in illness.

Specific Types of Intervention and Times Used to Select for Behavior Change Interventions, Individual Counseling

Codes		Time
99406	Smoking/tobacco use cessation	Intermediate – greater than 3 minutes up to 10 minutes
99407	Smoking/tobacco use cessation	Intensive – greater than 10 minutes
99408	Alcohol and/or substance abuse screening and intervention	Brief – 15 to 30 minutes
99409	Alcohol and/or substance abuse screening and intervention	Greater than 30 minutes

Behavior Change Interventions, Individual Counseling (99406-99409)

GENERAL GUIDELINES
These codes involve specific, validated intervention by:
- Assessing patient's readiness for change and barriers to change.
- Advising a change in patient's behavior.
- Providing specific suggested actions and motivational counseling.
- Arranging for services and follow-up.

Behavior change interventions may be provided:
- As part of treatment of condition(s) related to or potentially exacerbated by behavior.
- To change harmful behavior that has not yet resulted in illness.

No history or examination is required.

These codes are used for individual counseling for behavior change interventions.

For group counseling for patients with symptoms or established illness, see 99078.

These services are provided face-to-face with patient, using audio only or using audio-video telemedicine services if appropriate.

There are no separate codes for new and established patients or initial and subsequent services.

SELECTING CODES USING TIME OR MDM

These codes are reported using time only.

These are **NOT** add-on codes. Report one code based on total time spent providing the service.

Do **NOT** use these codes to report time spent in the intervention when the same time is also part of any other E/M services provided at the same encounter.

(continued on next page)

PATIENTS
These are services for counseling patients with conditions/concerns listed above.
PROVIDERS
Services provided by physician or other qualified healthcare provider.
OTHER SERVICES
Services **NOT** included in these codes. Report separately if appropriate: • Other distinct services on same date. Report separately with a modifier 25.
Do **NOT** report these codes on the same day as: • Codes for health behavior assessment and intervention services (96156, 96158, 96159, 96164-96168, 96170, 96171).   Do **NOT** report: • Code 99406 with code 99407. • Code 99409 with code 99408.

125

1. When a physician performs an E/M preventive care service, the extent of the exam is determined by the:
   a. Patient's age
   b. Patient's gender
   c. Patient's gender and age

2. Which of the following is NOT true about preventive medicine codes:
   a. Documentation must include the patient's age
   b. Documentation must include whether the patient is new or established to this practice
   c. Codes include counseling if done
   d. All of these statements are true

3. Preventive medicine codes do **NOT** include:
   a. A comprehensive examination
   b. Counseling regarding risk factor reduction
   c. Routine vaccinations
   d. Ordering of lab tests

4. A preventive medicine service is provided:
   a. When the patient has a documented illness
   b. Only for infants
   c. At the same time as a diagnostic procedure
   d. When the patient is not sick

5. Counseling and risk factor reduction codes include:
   a. Examination
   b. Time
   c. Counseling only
   d. Ordering laboratory tests

6. Behavioral change intervention codes are **NOT** reported for:
   a. Smoking cessation counseling
   b. Alcohol abuse intervention counseling
   c. Substance abuse screening
   d. Group counseling for these behaviors

7. Which of these services include a comprehensive history and examination?
   a. Preventive care services
   b. Counseling and risk factor reduction
   c. Behavioral change intervention
   d. All of these services include a comprehensive history and examination

See Appendix B for quiz answers.

Chapter 12

CPT® Services Provided by Interdisciplinary Teams

Interdisciplinary teams provide:
- Medical Team Conferences (99366-99368)
- Care Plan Oversight (99374-99389)
- Transitional Care Management Services (99495, 99496)

These codes are reported for establishing, implementing, revising and monitoring a care plan for a specific patient.

For care management services (chronic and principal care management), see chapter 13. For mental health/behavioral care management, see chapter 14.

These codes do **NOT** require the specific elements of a care plan used with care management services codes (99424-+99427, +99437, +99439, 99487, +99489, 99490, 99491). See chapter 13.

Comparison of Services provided by Interdisciplinary Teams

Codes		Description of Services
99366-99368	Medical team conferences	Services performed by interdisciplinary team (at least 3 providers). Providers also perform face-to-face services outside conference visit. No medical decision making required.
99374-99380	Care plan oversight	Services performed by interdisciplinary team. Supervision of individuals in home health agency, hospice, or nursing facility. No medical decision making required.
99495, 99496	Transitional care management services	Services performed by interdisciplinary team in coordination with community service agencies. Patient is being transferred from an inpatient/observation or nursing facility setting to community setting. Requires moderate or high complexity medical decision making.

Each of these oversight and management codes are discussed in detail on the following pages.

Medical Team Conferences

These case management services involve a physician or other qualified healthcare professional. The provider is responsible for directing care of a patient and coordinating, managing access to, initiating, and/or supervising other health care services needed by the patient.

These codes are selected by the provider and whether or not the patient is present.

The Center for Medicare and Medicaid Services (CMS) considers these services bundled into payment for other services and will not reimburse for them separately.

Summary of Criteria Used to Select Medical Team Conferences Codes

Code	Providers	Patient and/or family	Time in a calendar month
99366	Non-physician health care provider	Present	30 minutes or more
99367	Physician	Not present	30 minutes or more
99368	Nonphysician health care provider	Not present	30 minutes or more

Guidelines - Medical Team Conferences (99366-99368)

GENERAL GUIDELINES
An interdisciplinary team conference develops, coordinates and implements services for a specific patient. The providers may meet with: Patient   Surrogate decision maker(s) (eg, legal guardian) Family member(s)   Caregiver(s) There are no separate codes for new and established patients or initial and subsequent services. Codes are selected using time only.
Use code 99366 if: • Services are provided by nonphysicians; and • the patient is present for any part of the conference.
Use code 99367 if: • Services are provided by physicians; and • patient is not present. If services are provided by a physician and the patient and/or family is present, use other E/M codes using time to determine the level of service. Do **NOT** use code 99367.
Use code 99368 if: • Services are provided by nonphysicians; and • Patient is not present

(continued on next page)

SELECTING CODES USING TIME OR MDM

These codes are selected using time only.

Time in minutes within a calendar month:
- Must be at least 30 minutes.
- Begins with review of an individual patient.
- Ends at conclusion of review.
- Not limited to time that the participant is personally communicating with other team members, patient or family
- Reporting participant must be present for all time reported.

Do **NOT** report these codes if time:
- Was less than 30 minutes.
- Was spent in record keeping or generating a report.

PATIENTS

Use code 99366 if patient is present for all or part of conference.

Use codes 99367, 99368 if patient is **NOT** present for conference.

PROVIDERS

Providers may be physicians, other qualified healthcare professionals or non-physician providers.

Non-physician providers include:

Speech/language pathologists	Physician assistants	Physical therapists
Audiologists	Geneticists	Psychologists
Occupational therapists	Pharmacists	Social workers
Registered dietitians	Genetic counselors	

Providers in conference:
- Minimum of 3 providers from different specialties or disciplines.
- Only one member of the same specialty can report these codes. Other participants of same specialty should use E/M codes with time as the controlling factor.
- Must be actively involved in development, revision, coordination and implementation of health care services needed by patient.

Provider reporting these codes must perform these services:
- Before the conference - Face-to-face evaluation or treatment of the patient, within last 60 days.
- During the conference – Document their participation, contributed information, and subsequent treatment recommendations made. Provider must be present for all time being reporting.
- After the conference - Be directly involved with the patient, providing face-to-face evaluation of treatments of the patient.

(continued on next page)

Guidelines - Medical Team Conferences (continued)

OTHER SERVICES

Do **NOT** include time spent providing the following services in time spent in a medical conference:
- Care plan oversight (99374, 99375, 99377-99380) provided during the same month.
- Prolonged services on date other than face-to-face service (99358, +99359).
- Psychotherapy (90832-90834, 90836-90840, 90846, 90847, 90849, 90853).
- Any other E/M service.

Do **NOT** report these codes during the same month as:
- Care management services (+99437, +99439, 99487, +99489-99491).

Do **NOT** report these codes:
- If physician performs face-to-face service with patient and/or family present on this date. Use other E/M codes based on time when counseling and/or coordination of care dominates encounter.
- If provider's participation in the conference is due to a contract with an organization or facility.

Care Plan Oversight Services

These codes are reported for care plan oversight for patients in specific locations. The patient is not present during the oversight service.

Codes are selected by patient's location and total time within a calendar month.

Summary of Criteria Used to Select Care Plan Oversight Codes

Codes		Patient Location	Time
99374	Care plan oversight	Patient in home, domiciliary or equivalent environment, or Alzheimer's facility Care provided by home health agency	15-29 minutes within a calendar month
99375	Care plan oversight	Patient in home, domiciliary or equivalent environment, or Alzheimer's facility Care provided by home health agency	30 minutes or more within a calendar month
99377	Care plan oversight	Patient in hospice care	15-29 minutes within a calendar month
99378	Care plan oversight	Patient in hospice care	30 minutes within a calendar month
99379	Care plan oversight	Patient in nursing facility	15-29 minutes within a calendar month
99380	Care plan oversight	Patient in nursing facility	30 minutes within a calendar month

Note: codes 99375, 99378, 99380 are **NOT** add-on codes. Select a code by total time spent in providing the service.

131

Guidelines - Care Plan Oversight (99374, 99375, 99377-99380)

GENERAL GUIDELINES

Services include:
- Oversight of complex and multidisciplinary care modalities for patient.
- Regular development and/or revision of care plan.
- Review of subsequent reports of patient status.
- Review of related laboratory and other studies.
- Communication (including telephone calls) with others involved in assessment or care decisions, including:
  - Health care professional(s).
  - Family member(s).
  - Surrogate decision maker(s) (eg, legal guardian).
  - Key caregiver(s).
- Integration of new information into the medical treatment plan.
- Adjustment of medical therapy as needed.

These services are reported for non-face-to-face services (patient not present).

There are no separate codes for new or established patients or initial or subsequent service.

Codes are selected using patient location and time within a calendar month.

SELECTING CODES USING TIME OR MDM

These services are reported by minutes within a calendar month.

PATIENTS

Patient **NOT** present during service.
Patient may be located in home health agency, hospice, or nursing facility.

PROVIDERS

Codes do not specify that services must be provided by physician, other qualified health care professional or other individual.

Only one individual may report these codes for a given time period.

OTHER SERVICES

Services **NOT** included in these codes. Report separately if appropriate:
- E/M service for office/outpatient services, hospital, home or residence, nursing facility, or domiciliary or non-face-to-face services.

Do **NOT** report these codes if the patient was present during service.

Do **NOT** report these codes if service provided during the same service time as:
- Telephone services provided by non-physician (98966-98968).
- Telephone services provided by physician (99441-99443).
- Online digital E/M services (99421-99423).
- Service provided with complex chronic care management services (99487-+99489).

Do **NOT** report these codes for:
- More than one location during the same month.
- Supervision of patients in nursing facility or under care of home health agencies UNLESS the patient requires recurrent supervision of therapy.
- Provider's work is of very low intensity or requires only infrequent supervision. This is included in the pre- and post-encounter work included in home, office/outpatient and nursing facility or residence codes.

Transitional Care Management Services (TCM)

Transitional care management services are provided during patient's transition from an inpatient setting to a community setting. The patient has medical and/or psychosocial problems that require a moderate or high level of MDM.

These services include coordination of care performed by providers representing multiple disciplines and community service agencies. The services may be provided by a physician, other qualified healthcare professional, and/or clinical staff. See next page for a description of services that can be provided by each.

Services include both one face-to-face encounter with patient and subsequent non-face-to-face encounters. Code depends on the level of medical decision making and date of first face-to-face communication.

Summary of Criteria Used to Select Transitional Care Management Codes

Codes		Medical Decision Making**	Face-to-face visit
99495	Communication* with the patient and/or caregiver within 2 business days of discharge.	At least moderate complexity	Within 7 calendar days
		Moderate or High complexity	Within 8-14 calendar days
99496	Communication* with the patient and/or caregiver within 2 business days of discharge.	High complexity	Within 7 calendars days

*First communication may be direct contact (face-to-face services with patient), by telephone or by electronic means.
**The level of MDM is determined by the medical decision making over the period of the service (30 days).

These services include patient transfer from one setting to another. For example:

Patient transferred FROM	Patient transferred TO
Inpatient hospital setting – including: • Acute hospital • Rehabilitation hospital • Long-term acute care hospital • Partial hospital • Observation status in a hospital • Skilled nursing facility/nursing facility	These settings: • Home* • Domiciliary • Rest home or • Assisted living. • Group home**

*Home may be defined as a private residence, temporary lodging, or short-term accommodation (eg, hotel, campground, hostel or cruise ship).

Use these codes for patients transferred to a group home that is **NOT licensed as an intermediate care facility for individuals with intellectual disabilities, custodial care facility or residential substance abuse treatment facility.

Services may be provided by a physician and/or other qualified health care professional and/or clinical staff. Each provider performs different non-face-to-face services as described below.

Transitional Care Management Services (TCM) (99495, 99496)
Providers – NON-FACE-TO-FACE Services

Services provided by CLINICAL STAFF under supervision of Physician/QHP	Services provided by PHYSICIAN OR OTHER QUALIFIED HEALTH CARE PROFESSIONAL
Assessment of Patient's Treatment and Condition	
Assessment and support for patient/caregiver's adherence to treatment and medication regimes.	Obtaining and reviewing discharge information such as: • Discharge summary, as available, or • Continuity of care documents. Reviewing need for follow-up on pending diagnostic tests and treatments.
Communication	
Communication regarding aspects of care with: • Patient • Family members • Guardian or caretaker • Surrogate decision makers • Other professionals regarding aspects of care.	Communication with: • Other qualified health care professionals who will assume or reassume care of patient's system-specific problems.
Education	
Education provided to patient and/or family/caretaker to support: • Patient's self-management • Independent living • Activities of daily living	Education of: • Patient • Family • Guardian • Caregiver
Community Resources	
Identification of available community and health resources. Communication with: • Home health agencies and • Other community services utilized by the patient.	Establishment or reestablishment of referrals. Arranging for needed community resources.
Facilitating access to care and services needed by the patient and/or family.	Assistance in scheduling any required follow-up with community providers and services.

Guidelines - Transitional Care Management Services (TCM) (99495. 99496)

GENERAL GUIDELINES

Services address any needed coordination of care between providers and community service agencies.

Reporting individual provides or oversees management and/or coordination of services, as needed, for:
- All medical conditions
- Psychosocial needs
- Activities of daily living support.

Documentation must include:
- Timing of initial post-discharge communication with patient or caregiver
- Date of the face-to-face visit with patient
- Complexity of medical decision making.

Code depends on when face-to-face encounter with patient took place and level of MDM.

There are no separate codes for new or established patient or initial or subsequent service.

SELECTING CODES USING TIME OR MDM

Codes are selected using number of days since discharge and medical decision making.

Medical decision making must be moderate or high.

Time begins on date of patient's discharge from facility and continues for next 29 days.

Code 99495 –
- Face-to-face visit within 7 days of discharge. MDM must be moderate complexity or higher.
- Face-to-face visit within 8-14 days of discharge. MDM must be moderate complexity or higher.

Code 99496 –
- Face-to-face visit within 7 calendar days of discharge from facility. MDM is high complexity.

PATIENTS

Patient is being transferred from hospital setting to home, domiciliary, rest home or assisted living setting.

Patient communicates with provider following discharge from inpatient setting.

Patient has medical and/or psychosocial problems that require moderate or high complexity medical decision making during transitions in care.

(continued on next page)

135

PROVIDERS

See page 132 for a list of non-face-to-face services provided by physicians and clinical staff.

Provider may initiate first communication with patient either face-to-face with patient or by telephone or electronic means.

Face-face service must be with specified number of days after discharge. See times listed in section above on selecting codes.

Services provided by:
- Licensed clinical staff under direction of physician or other qualified health care professional.
- Physician or other qualified health care professional.

Codes reported by:
- Only one individual.
- Once within 30 days of discharge.

Others involved in providing these services should report other E/M codes.

See page 134 for a list of non-face-to-face services by clinical staff and physician/QHP.

OTHER SERVICES

Services **NOT** included in these codes. Report separately if appropriate:
- Hospital or observation discharge services. Discharge service cannot be counted as initial face-to-face visit with patient for these services.
- Additional E/M services provided on subsequent dates after first face-to-face visit.
- General behavioral health integration care management (99484).
- Remote physiologic monitoring treatment management services (99457, +99458).

Do **NOT** report these codes during the same period as:
- Online digital E/M during same time period (99421-99423).
- Telephone services (99441-99443).
- Chronic care management if services are separate (+99437, +99439, 99487, +99489, 99491).
- A postoperative period.

A decision tree on the next page describes coding for transitional care management services.

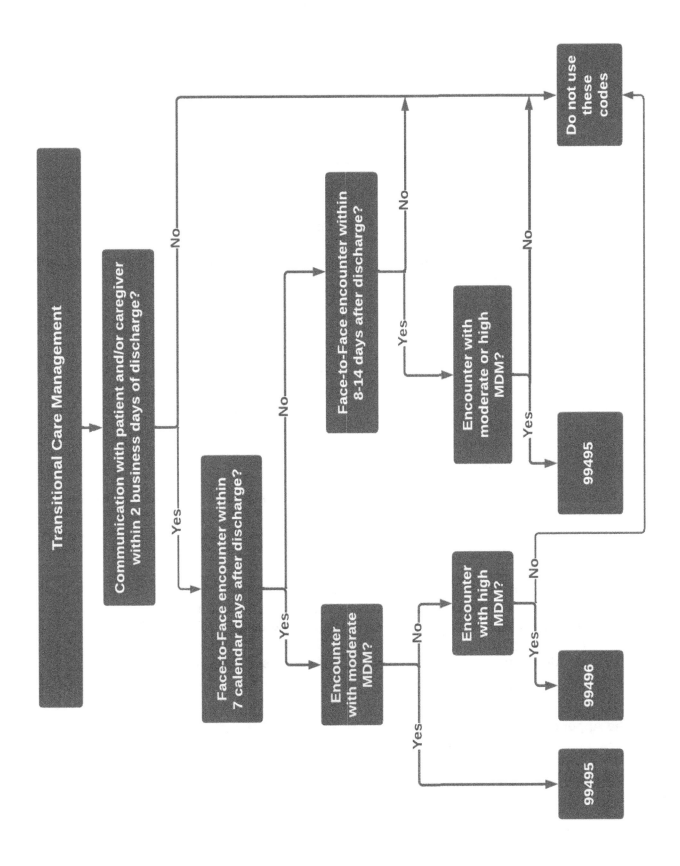

Transitional Care Management

Communication with patient and/or caregiver within 2 business days of discharge?

- Yes → Face-to-Face encounter within 7 calendar days after discharge?
  - Yes → Encounter with moderate MDM?
    - Yes → 99495
    - No → Encounter with high MDM?
      - Yes → 99496
      - No → Do not use these codes
  - No → Face-to-Face encounter within 8-14 days after discharge?
    - Yes → Encounter with moderate or high MDM?
      - Yes → 99495
      - No → Do not use these codes
    - No → Do not use these codes
- No → Do not use these codes

137

1. Care plan oversight services are reported by time:
    a. Per day
    b. Per month
    c. In minutes

2. Transitional care management codes are selected based on:
    a. Calendar days since face-to-face visit
    b. Level of MDM
    c. Level of MDM and date of first face-to-face visit.
    d. Location patient is being transferred to
    e. Location patient is being transferred from

3. A patient in an Alzheimer's facility is receiving care plan oversight. The oversight is reported using these codes:
    a. 99374, 99375
    b. 99377, 99378
    c. 99379, 99380

4. Transitional care is provided to a patient after discharge. The service includes high complexity MDM and the provider reports code 99496. The first communication with the patient must occur:
    a. Within 7 calendar days of discharge
    b. Within 8 calendar days of discharge
    c. Within 14 calendar days of discharge

5. Medical team conferences that require presence of a physician is reported using code:
    a. 99366
    b. 99367
    c. 99368

6. A medical team conference requires at least:
    a. Minimum of 3 providers from different specialties or disciplines.
    b. Minimum of 3 providers from same specialty or disciplines.
    c. Only 1 provider
    d. Minimum of 4 providers from same or different specialties or disciplines.

See Appendix B for quiz answers.

Chapter 13

CPT® Care Management Services

Care management services are reported for establishing, implementing, revising and monitoring a care plan for a specific patient.

Care management services include these code categories:
- Chronic Care Management Services (99490, 99491, +99437, +99439)
- Complex Care Management (99487, +99489)
- Principal Care Management (99424-+99427)

Each of these categories include care planning. There are no separate codes for this planning; the planning is included in the codes for principal care, chronic care, and complex chronic care management. See page 143.

For mental health/behavioral care management, see chapter 14.

For care management services (chronic and principal care management), see chapter 12.

These codes provide management and support services to a patient. Different sets of codes are used to report different types of care management services:

Summary of Criteria Used to Select Care Management Codes

Codes		Correct Code Determined by -		
		Medically appropriate history and/or examination	MDM	Time
99424-+99427	Principal care management services			√
+99437, +99439 99490, 99491	Chronic care management services			√
99487, +99489	Complex chronic care management services		Moderate or High	√

The next pages discuss general guidelines for care plan management codes. These are applicable to principal care, chronic care, and complex chronic care management codes. These pages include:
- General guidelines.
- Requirements for office/practice personnel reporting these codes.
- Components of a care plan.
- Requirements for each category of care management services.

Guidelines - Care Plan Management Services
(99424-+99427, +99437, +99439, 99490, 99491, 99487, +99489)

GENERAL GUIDELINES

The goal of care management services is to:
- Improve care coordination.
- Reduce avoidable hospital services.
- Improve patient engagement.
- Decrease care fragmentation.

Services include the work to:
- Establish, implement, revise or monitor the care plan.
- Coordinate the care of other professionals and agencies.
- Educate the patient or caregiver about the patient's condition, care plan and prognosis.

Services may be face-to-face with patient or non-face-to-face.

There are no separate codes for new or established patients or initial or subsequent service.

See page 141 for a discussion of requirements for office personnel providing these services.

SELECTING CODES USING TIME OR MDM

Codes are selected using time and medical decision making. Time is measured in minutes within a calendar month.

Clinical staff and physician/other healthcare professionals may provide distinct services to the same patient at different time. Each can report their time separately.

Do **NOT** count any time and activities in care plan management for time used for another reported service.

PATIENTS

The patient may be residing at home or in a domiciliary, rest home, or assisted living facility.

PROVIDERS

These services may be provided by:
- Clinical staff, under direction of physician or other qualified health care professional, OR
- A physician or other qualified health care professional who oversees activities of the care team.

All care team members must be clinically integrated.

Do **NOT** report care management codes for a surgeon who is also providing care during a post-operative period.

See page 141 for detailed discussion of provider services included in these codes.

(continued on next page)

Office/Practice Setting Personnel
Must Be Able To Provide These Services

IDENTIFY/INITIATE CARE MANAGEMENT

Office/practice personnel must:

- Use a standardized methodology to identify patients who require care management services.

- Have an internal care management process/function whereby a patient identified as meeting the requirements for these services starts receiving them in a timely manner.

MAINTAIN RECORD KEEPING

Record keeping must:

- Include an electronic health record system so that care providers have timely access to clinical information.

- Include ability to document and share an electronic and/or printed plan of care with the patient and/or caregiver.

- Use a form and format in the medical record that is standardized within the practice.

PROVIDE COMMUNICATION BETWEEN PATIENT OR CAREGIVER AND PROVIDER

Providers must be able to:

- Provide patient/caregivers a means to contact health care professionals in the practice to address urgent needs regardless of the time of day or day of the week (24/7).

- Communicate and engage with patient, family members, guardian or caretaker, surrogate decision makers, and/or other professionals regarding aspects of patient's care.

- Educate patient and/or family/caregiver to support patient's self-management, independent living, and activities of daily living.

PROVIDE CONTINUITY AND COORDINATION OF CARE

Providers must be able to:

- Provide continuity of care with a designated member of the care team for scheduling successive routine appointments.

- Be able to coordinate care among all service providers as appropriate for each patient.

- Provide timely access and management for follow-up after an emergency department visit or facility discharge.

- Develop care plan to meet needs of the specific patient.*

*Requirements for the care plan are discussed beginning on page 143.

(continued on next page)

141

Guidelines - Care Plan Management Services (continued)

Office/Practice Setting Personnel
Must Be Able To Provide These Services (continued)

TREATMENT/DATA COLLECTION SERVICES
Providers must be able to: • Collect health outcomes data and document as appropriate in patient registries. • Assess and support patient/caregiver's adherence to treatment and medication regimes • Provide ongoing review of patient status, including review of laboratory and other studies not reported as part of another E/M service. • Develop, communicate and maintain a comprehensive care plan. • Facilitate access to care and services needed by patient and/or family. • Manage transitions between types/locations of care that are not reported with transitional care management codes (99495, 99496).
SERVICES RELATED TO COMMUNITY RESOURCES/ACCESS TO CARE
Providers must be able to: • Communicate with home health agencies and other community services used by patient. • Identify available community and health resources.

CPT© codes and descriptions only copyright 2023 American Medical Association. All right reserved.
Other content copyright Medical Coding Made Easy LLC © 2023 All Rights Reserved.

Guidelines – Care Planning

Care planning does **NOT** have its own set of codes. Planning is included in the other care management services codes discussed in this chapter.

GENERAL GUIDELINES
A plan of care is: • Based on a physical, mental, cognitive, social, functional, and environmental evaluation of the patient.   • Provides a simple and concise overview of the patient and his or her medical conditions.   • Contains useful documents for patients, caregivers, health care professionals and others, as necessary.   • Developed for care management services.   • Includes specific goals for each condition; goals should be achievable and time specific when possible.   • Be relevant to patient's well-being and lifestyle.   Care planning should be: • Updated periodically based on status or goal changes.   • Revised as needed, but at least annually.   • Shared with patient and/or caregiver in electronic or printed format.

COMPONENTS OF A TYPICAL PLAN OF CARE*	
• A problem list. • Expected outcome and prognosis. • Measurable treatment goals. • Cognitive assessment. • Functional assessment. • Symptom management.	• Planned interventions. • Medical management. • Environmental evaluation. • Caregiver assessment. • Interaction and coordination with outside resources and health care professionals and others, as necessary. • Summary of advanced directives.

*These elements are a guide to development of a meaningful plan for a specific patient's needs, not a strict set of requirements. Each should be addressed as appropriate for a specific patient.

The following pages describe these care plan management categories in detail:
• Principal care management
• Chronic care management
• Complex chronic care management

Each type of care plan management includes the requirements listed on pages 140-142 and development of a care plan.

See page 153 for a comparison of these different types of care plan management services.

Principal Care Management

Care management services are provided to patients with one high-risk disease which is expected to last at least 3 months. Codes are selected by time and the provider.

Summary of Criteria Used to Select Principal Care Management Codes

Codes		Medical Decision Making	Time	Provider
99424	Principal care management for a single, high-risk disease		First 30 minutes	Physician or other QHP
+99425	Principal care management for a single, high-risk disease		Each additional 30 minutes	Physician or other QHP
99426	Principal care management for a single, high-risk disease		First 30 minutes	Clinical staff directed by physician or other QHP
+99427	Principal care management for a single, high-risk disease		Each additional 30 minutes	Clinical staff directed by physician or other QHP

Guidelines – Principal Care Management (99424-+99427)

GENERAL GUIDELINES

Condition requires management services to:

- Develop, establish, implement, revise or monitor a care plan specific to a single disease.
- Make frequent adjustments to the medication regimen and/or the management of the condition due to its complexity and comorbidities.
- Provide ongoing communication and care coordination between all practitioners who are furnishing care.

Includes care planning. See requirements on page 143.

These services are provided face-to-face with patient or non-face-to-face.

There are no separate codes for new or established patients or initial or subsequent service.

(continued on next page)

Guidelines – Principal Care Management (continued)

SELECTING CODES USING TIME OR MDM

Codes are selected by type of provider and minutes within a calendar month.

No specific level of medical decision making is included.

Do **NOT** report these codes if total time in a calendar month is less than 30 minutes.

Services personally provided **by physician/other health care professional** in a calendar month:
- 99424 – First 30 minutes. Report code once per calendar month.
- +99425 – Each additional 30 minutes. This code can be reported in multiple units when appropriate in a calendar month.

Sometimes services are provided <u>personally</u> by the treating physician/other qualified health care professional AND by clinical staff. In these cases:
- Do **NOT** report codes both for clinical staff services (99426, +99427) and physicians/other qualified healthcare professionals services (99424, +99425) during same calendar month.
- Add physician's time to clinical staff time to calculate total time. Report codes 99426, +99427. The physician's services and clinical staff services cannot be reported separately.

Services provided by **clinical staff** and directed by physician/other qualified health care professional:
- 99426 – First 30 minutes. Report once per calendar month.
- +99427 – Each additional 30 minutes. Report no more than twice per calendar month.

Clinical staff time includes time spent face-to-face with patient and non-face-to-face time with patient and/or family/caregivers/other professionals and agencies.

Do **NOT** count time of clinical staff on the day of an initial visit, which includes creation of care plan, initial explanation to the patient and/or caregiver, and obtaining consent.

PATIENTS

Patient has a single complex (high risk) chronic condition expected to last at least 3 months.

Sometimes a patient may have multiple chronic conditions that are severe enough to warrant complex chronic care management BUT this provider is performing only principal care management (addressing a single disease rather than the multiple conditions). Report a principal care management code only.

PROVIDERS

See also section above on Selecting Codes Using time or MDM.

Services may be provided by clinical staff (99426, +99427) or a physician/other health care professional (99424, +99425).

These codes can be reported by different providers in the same month for the same patient.

Documentation should reflect coordination among the different providers.

Services provided by clinical staff (99426, +99427) include:
- Face-to-face encounter with patient and/or non-face-to-face services.
- Communicating with patient and/or family, caregivers, other professionals and agencies.
- Creating, revising, documenting, and implementing the care plan.
- Teaching self-management to the patient.

(continued on next page)

OTHER SERVICES

These codes are **NOT** included in the principal care management codes. Report separately if appropriate:

- Behavioral or psychiatric collaborative care management services (99484, 99492, 99493, +99494).

Do **NOT** report these codes in the <u>same calendar month</u> as:

- End-stage renal disease services (90951-90970).
- Care plan oversight (99374, 99375, 99377-99380).
- Chronic care management (+99437, +99439, 99340, 99487, +99489-99491).
- Medication therapy management (99605-99607).

Do **NOT** report these codes for services provided during the <u>same service time</u> as:

- INR Monitoring services (93792, 93793).
- Patient education and training (98960-98962, 99071, 99078, 99080).
- Telephone services (98966-98968, 99441-99443).
- Online digital assessment/management (98970-98972).
- Analysis of data (99091).
- Prolonged services on date other than face-to-face service (99358, +99359).
- Medical team conference (99366-99368).
- Online digital E/M services (99421-99423).
- Medication therapy management (99605-99607).

Chronic Care Management

Chronic care management services are provided to patients with two or more chronic conditions expected to last at least 12 months or until death of patient. Codes are selected by provider and time.

Summary of Criteria Used to Select Chronic Care Management Codes

Codes		Medical Decision Making	Time	Provider
99490	Chronic care management for 2 or more chronic conditions Expected to last at least 3 months		First 20 minutes	Clinical staff directed by physician or other QHP
+99439	Chronic care management for 2 or more chronic conditions Expected to last at least 3 months		Each additional 20 minutes	Clinical staff directed by physician or other QHP
99491	Chronic care management for 2 or more chronic conditions Expected to last at least 3 months		First 30 minutes	Physician or other QHP
+99437	Chronic care management for 2 or more chronic conditions Expected to last at least 3 months		Each additional 30 minutes	Physician or other QHP

Guidelines – Chronic Care Management (99490, 99491, +99437, +99439)

GENERAL GUIDELINES

These services address, as needed, all medical conditions, psychosocial needs and activities of daily living for a specific patient.

Includes care planning. See requirements on page 143.

Services provided face-to-face with patient or non-face-to-face.

There are no separate codes for new or established patients or initial or subsequent service.

SELECTING CODES USING TIME OR MDM

These codes are reported using minutes within a calendar month.

No specific level of medical decision making is included.

Do **NOT** report these codes if total time in a calendar month is less than 20 minutes.

If chronic care services last 60 minutes or more and include moderate or high complexity medical decision, use complex chronic care management codes (99487, +99489) instead of these chronic care management codes.

Services provided personally by **physician/other health care professional** -
- 99491 – First 30 minutes of care. Report code once per calendar month.
- +99437 – Each additional 20 minutes. This code can be reported in multiple units when appropriate.

Sometimes services are provided <u>personally</u> by both the treating physician/other qualified health care professional and by clinical staff. In these cases:
- Do **NOT** report both clinical staff services (99490, +99439) and physician/other qualified health care professional services (99491) in the same month.

Add physician's time to clinical staff time to calculate total time. Report codes 99490, +99439. The physician's services and clinical staff services cannot be reported separately.

Services provided by **clinical staff** under supervision of physician/qualified health care provider:
- 99490 – Report code once per calendar month. First 30 minutes of care.
- +99439 – Report no more than twice per calendar month. Each additional 20 minutes.

Do **NOT** count time of clinical staff on the day of an initiating visit, which includes creation of care plan, initial explanation to the patient and/or caregiver, and obtaining consent.

PATIENTS

Patient has:
- Chronic conditions that places them at significant risk of death, acute exacerbation/ decompensation or functional decline.
- Two or more chronic continuous or episodic conditions expected to last 12 months or until patient's death.
- Medical and/or psychosocial needs that require establishing, implementing, revising or monitoring a care plan.

(continued on next page)

PROVIDERS

See also section on previous page on Selecting Codes Using Time or MDM.

Use codes 99491, +99437 if services provided by a <u>physician/other QHP</u>.

Use codes 99490, +99439 if services provided by <u>clinical staff</u> directed by a physician or other QHP.

Services provided by <u>clinical staff</u> include:
- Services face-to-face with patient and/or non-face-to-face.
- Communicating with patient and/or family, caregivers, other professionals and agencies.
- Creating, revising, documenting, and implementing the care plan.
- Teaching self-management to the patient.

MULTIPLE SERVICES

A provider may perform a face-to-face E/M code with the patient and/or family on the same date as chronic care management.
- Report 99347, 99491 in addition to the chronic care codes.

Do **NOT** include time spent providing the other E/M service in calculating the time used for chronic care management.

OTHER SERVICES

These codes are **NOT** included in the chronic care management codes. Report separately if appropriate:
- Behavioral or psychiatric collaborative care management services (99484, 99492, 99293, +99494).

Do **NOT** report chronic care management codes provided during the <u>same service time</u> as:
- INR monitoring services (93792, 93793).
- Online digital assessment/management (98970-98972).
- Education and training (98960, 98961, 98962, 99071, 99078).
- Preparation of special reports (99080).
- Analysis of data (99091).
- Prolonged services on date other than face-to-face service (99358, +99359).
- Medical team conference (99366-99368).
- Online digital E/M services (99421-99423).
- Telephone services (98966-98968, 99441-99443).
- Medication therapy management services (99605-99607).

Do **NOT** report +99437, +99439, 99490, 99491 in the <u>same calendar month</u> with:
- End-stage renal disease services during same calendar month (90951-90970).
- Care plan oversight (99374, 99375, 99377-99380).
- Principal care management (99424-+99427).
- Complex chronic care management (99487, +99489, 99491).
- Medication therapy management services (99605-99607).

Do **NOT** report +99437, 99491 in <u>same calendar month</u> with:
- Transitional care management (99495-99496).

Do **NOT** report +99439, 99490 in the <u>same calendar month</u> with:
- Principal care management (99424-+99427).
- Chronic care management (99490).

149

Complex Chronic Care Management

These codes are reported for chronic care management services for patients with two or more chronic conditions expected to last at least 12 months or until patient's death. Services are provided by clinical staff. Moderate or high complexity MDM is required.

Summary of Criteria Used to Select Complex Chronic Care Management Codes

Codes		Medical Decision Making	Time	Provider
99487	Chronic care management for 2 or more chronic conditions or until patient's death	Moderate or high	First 60 minutes	Clinical staff directed by physician or other QHP
+99489	Chronic care management for 2 or more chronic conditions or until patient's death	Moderate or high	Each additional 30 minutes	Clinical staff directed by physician or other QHP

Guidelines – Complex Chronic Care Management (99487, +99489)

GENERAL GUIDELINES
These services address, as needed, all medical conditions, psychosocial needs and activities of daily living of the patient.
Includes care planning. See requirements on page 143.
Services may be face-to-face with patient or non-face-to-face.
There are no separate codes for new or established patients or initial or subsequent service.

SELECTING CODES USING TIME OR MDM
Codes are selected using time within a calendar month and medical decision making.
MDM must be at least moderate complexity.
Clinical staff time must be at least 60 minutes.
99487 – First 60 minutes in a calendar month. +99489 – Each additional 30 minutes. May be reported in multiple units if appropriate.
Do **NOT** report clinical staff time on the day of an initiating visit, which includes creation of care plan, initial explanation to the patient and/or caregiver, and obtaining consent.
Sometimes the service is provided <u>personally</u> by both the treating physician/other qualified health care professional and by clinical staff. In these cases: • Do **NOT** report codes for both clinical staff services and physician/other qualified health care provider during the same calendar month. • Add physician's time to clinical staff time to calculate total time. Report codes 99487, +99489. The physician's services and clinical staff services cannot be reported separately.

(Continued on next page)

PATIENTS

Patient:
- Has chronic conditions that place them at significant risk of death, acute exacerbation/decompensation or functional decline.
- Has two or more chronic continuous or episodic conditions expected to last 12 months or until patient's death.
- Needs complex chronic care management identified by practice-specific or other published algorithms.

Patients may:
- Have multiple complex diseases and morbidities.
- Use multiple medications.
- Be unable to perform activities of daily living.
- Require a caregiver.
- Have had repeated admissions or emergency department visits.
- Need coordination between a number of different specialties and services.
- Have cognitive impairment that may result in poor compliance with treatment plan; substantial assistance from a caregiver needed.
- Have psychiatric and other medical comorbidities (eg, dementia and chronic obstructive pulmonary diseases or substance abuse and diabetes) that complicate care.
- Require social support.
- Have difficulty accessing care.

Typical **adult** patients:
- Are being treated with three or more prescription medications.
- May be receiving other types of therapeutic interventions (eg, physical therapy or occupational therapy).

Typical **pediatric** patients:
- Receive three or more therapeutic interventions (eg, medication, nutritional support, respiratory therapy).

PROVIDERS

See also section on previous page on Selecting Codes Using time or MDM.

Services provided by clinical staff, either face-to-face with patient or non-face-to-face.

Clinical staff are directed by physician or other QHP.

Services include:
- Communicating with patient and/or family, caregivers, other professionals and agencies.
- Creating, revising, documenting, and implementing the care plan.
- Teaching self-management to the patient.

Report codes for services by one provider for a calendar month.

(continued on next page)

OTHER SERVICES
These codes are **NOT** included in the complex chronic care management codes. Report separately if appropriate: • Behavioral or psychiatric collaborative care management services (99484, 99492, 99493, +99494).
Do **NOT** report these services with the complex chronic care management services during <u>same calendar month</u>: • End-stage renal disease services during same calendar month (90951-90970). • Oversight services (99374-99380). • Principal care management services (99424, +99427). • Care plan oversight services (99374, 99375, 99377-99380). • Principal care management services (+99437, +99439). • Chronic care management services (99490, 99491). Do **NOT** report complex chronic services using same <u>service time</u> for these other codes: • INR monitoring services (93792, 93793). • Education and training (98960-98962, 99071, 99078). • Telephone services (98966-98968, 99441-99443). • Online digital assessment/management (98970-98972). • Preparation of special reports (99080). • Analysis of data (99091). • Prolonged services on date other than face-to-face service (99358, +99359). • Medical team conference (99366-99368). • Online digital E/M services (99421-99423). • Medication therapy management services (99605-99607).

A comparison of these care management codes is on the following page.

Comparison – Care Management Codes

These codes are selected by number of chronic conditions, who is providing the service, and time.

Codes	Description	Minutes in a calendar month	Provider
Chronic Care Management			
99490	2 or more chronic conditions Expected to last 12 months or until patient's death No MDM specified.	20 minutes	Clinical staff supervised by physician or other QHP
+99439	2 or more chronic conditions Expected to last 12 months or until patient's death No MDM specified.	Each additional 20 minutes	Clinical staff supervised by physician or other QHP
99491	2 or more chronic conditions Expected to last 12 months or until patient's death No MDM specified.	30 minutes	Physician or other QHP
+99437	2 or more chronic conditions Expected to last 12 months or until patient's death No MDM specified.	Each additional 30 minutes	Physician or other QHP
Complex Chronic Care Management			
99487	2 or more chronic conditions Expected to last 12 months or until patient's death Requires moderate or high MDM	60 minutes	Physician or other QHP
+99489	2 or more chronic conditions Expected to last 12 months or until patient's death Requires moderate or high MDM	Each additional 30 minutes	Physician or other QHP
Principal Care Management Services			
99424	1 complex chronic condition Expected to last at least 3 months No MDM specified.	30 minutes	Physician or other QHP
+99425	1 complex chronic condition Expected to last at least 3 months No MDM specified.	Each additional 30 minutes	Physician or other QHP
99426	1 complex chronic condition Expected to last at least 3 months No MDM specified.	30 minutes	Clinical staff supervised by physician or other QHP
+99427	1 complex chronic condition Expected to last at least 3 months No MDM specified.	Each additional 30 minutes	Clinical staff supervised by physician or other QHP

A decision tree on the next page describes coding for care management services codes.

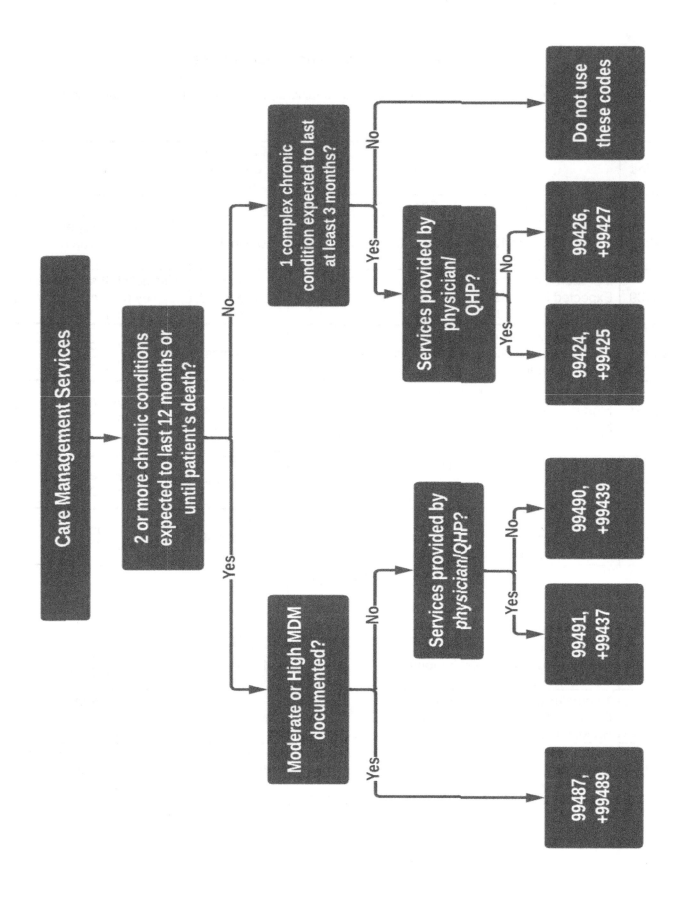

Care Management Services

2 or more chronic conditions expected to last 12 months or until patient's death?

No → 1 complex chronic condition expected to last at least 3 months?

- **No →** Do not use these codes
- **Yes →** Services provided by physician/QHP?
  - **No →** 99426, +99427
  - **Yes →** 99424, +99425

Yes → Moderate or High MDM documented?

- **No →** Services provided by physician/QHP?
  - **No →** 99490, +99439
  - **Yes →** 99491, +99437
- **Yes →** 99487, +99489

1. Care management services includes 3 categories. Which of the following do **NOT** include a separate category of codes:
    a. Chronic care management
    b. Complex chronic care management
    c. Principal care management
    d. Care planning

2. The difference between chronic care management codes and complex chronic care management codes is:
    a. The number of chronic conditions
    b. The time the conditions are expected to last
    c. Requirement for MDM

3. Principal care management codes 99426-+99427 can be reported by:
    a. Physicians only
    b. Qualified health care professionals only
    c. Clinical staff under supervision of physicians or qualified health care professional
    d. Physicians, qualified health care professionals or clinical staff

4. A specific level of MDM is required for:
    a. Chronic care management
    b. Complex chronic care management
    c. Principal care management
    d. Chronic care and complex chronic care management

5. Principal care services code +99427 can be reported:
    a. Once each calendar month
    b. As many times as appropriate during a calendar month
    c. Reported no more than twice per calendar month.

6. Care planning should be updated/revised:
    a. At least annually.
    b. Updated every month.
    c. Updated every week.

7. Do **NOT** report chronic care management codes +99437, 99491 with transitional care codes 99495-99496 within:
    a. 45 days
    b. The same calendar month
    c. The same calendar week
    d. The same 24 hours

156

Chapter 14

CPT® Behavioral/Mental Health Services

Behavioral/mental health services are for the care management services provided to patients with cognitive, behavior or psychiatric concerns.

These codes do **NOT** require the specific elements of a care plan used with care management services codes (99424, +99427, +99437, +99439, 99487, +99489, 99490, 99491). See chapter 13.

Codes are selected by time and provider.

Summary of Criteria Used to Select Behavioral/Mental Health Codes

Codes		Provider	Time
99483	Cognitive assessment and care plan services	Physician or other QHP	Typical time 60 minutes
99484	General behavioral health integration care management	Clinical staff directed by physician or other QHP	At least 20 minutes
99492	Psychiatric collaborative care management services	Consultant Physician or other QHP	Initial calendar month of care First 70 minutes
99493	Psychiatric collaborative care management services	Consultant Physician or other QHP	Subsequent calendar month of care First 60 minutes
+99494	Psychiatric collaborative care management services	Consultant Physician or other QHP	Initial or subsequent month of care Each additional 30 minutes

Each of these categories are discussed in detail in the following pages.

Cognitive Assessment and Care Plan Services

Cognitive assessment and care plan services include a comprehensive evaluation of a patient who exhibits signs and/or symptoms of cognitive impairment, including changes in memory, orientation and awareness.

Summary of Criteria Used to Select Cognitive Assessment and Care Plan Codes

Code		Medical Decision Making	Time
99483	Cognitive assessment and care plan services	Moderate or high	Typical time 60 minutes

Guidelines - Cognitive Assessment and Care Plan Services (99483)

GENERAL GUIDELINES

Services are performed to establish or confirm a diagnosis, etiology and severity of condition.
 	
 All the following services **MUST** be included:
 • Cognition-focused evaluation including a pertinent history and examination.
 • Medical decision making of moderate or high complexity. MDM includes assessing:
    ○ Current and likely progression of the disease.
    ○ The need to refer the patient for rehabilitative, social, legal, financial or community-based services.
    ○ The need for personal assistance services such as meals and transportation.
 • Functional assessment (e, basic and instrumental activities of daily living), including decision-making capacity.
 • Use of standardized instruments for staging of dementia (eg, functional assessment staging test [FAST], clinical dementia rating [DCR]).
 • Medication reconciliation (ensuring that prescribed medications match medications that the patient is actually taking).
 • Review of high-risk medications.
 • Evaluation for neuropsychiatric and behavioral symptoms, including depression, with use of standardized screening instrument(s).
 • Evaluation of patient's safety (eg, in their home or ability to drive a motor vehicle).
 • Identification of caregiver(s), and assessment of caregiver's knowledge, needs, social supports, and the willingness to take on caregiving tasks.
 • Development, updating, revision, or review of an advance care plan.
 • Creation of a written care plan, including initial plans to address any neuropsychiatric symptoms, neurocognitive symptoms, functional limitations, and need for referral to community resources (eg, rehabilitation services, adult day programs, support groups). Plan is shared with the patient and/or caregiver with initial education and support.
 	
 If **NOT** all of these services are provided or considered necessary, list appropriate E/M code instead of these cognitive assessment codes.
 	
 This code is reported for face-to-face encounters with patient.
 	
 There are no separate codes for new and established patients or initial and subsequent services.

(continued on next page)

SELECTING CODES USING TIME OR MDM

These codes are selected by time and medical decision making.

Level of medical decision **MUST** be moderate or high complexity.

No medically appropriate history and/or examination is required.

Typical time is 60 minutes.

Do **NOT** report this code more than once every 180 days.

The encounter may last longer than the typical time (60 minutes). If time is being used to select the level of service, use prolonged services code +99417. Code +99417 can be listed in multiple units when appropriate.

- For example, cognitive assessment and care plan services lasted a total of 75 minutes. List code 99483 (60 minutes) plus +99217 (additional 15 minutes).
- See Chapter 10 for more information on prolonged services.

PATIENTS

Patient has an indication of a cognitive impairment which may be due to:
- Psychoactive medications
- Chronic pain syndromes
- Infection
- Depression
- Other brain disease (eg, tumor, stroke, normal pressure hydrocephalus).

PROVIDERS

Services are provided by a physician or another qualified healthcare professional.

OTHER SERVICES

Do **NOT** report these codes with:
- Office or other outpatient services (99202-99205, 99211-99215)
- Consultations (99242-99245)
- Home or residence (99341-99350)
- Medical team conference (99366-99368)
- Advance care planning (99497, +99498)
- Psychiatric diagnostic procedures (90785, 90791, 90792)
- Brief emotional/behavioral assessment (96127)
- Psychological or neuropsychiatric or neuropsychological test administration (96146)
- Health risk assessment administration (96160, 96161)
- Medication therapy management services (99605, 99606, 99607)

General Behavioral Health Integration Care Management

General behavioral health integration care management services are provided by clinical staff to a patient with a behavioral health condition (including substance use) that requires care management services.

Summary of Specific Criteria Used to Select
General Behavior Health Integration Management Code

Codes		Medical Decision Making	Provider	Time
99484	General behavioral health integration management		Clinical staff under supervision of physician or other QHP	At least 20 minutes

General Behavioral Health Integration Care Management (99484)

GENERAL GUIDELINES

Services include:

- Initial assessment or follow-up monitoring, including use of applicable validated rating scales.

- Behavioral health care planning in relation to behavioral/psychiatric health problems, including revision of plan for patients who are not progressing or whose status has changed.

- Facilitating and coordinating treatment such as psychotherapy, pharmacotherapy, counseling and/or psychiatric consultation.

- Continuity of care with a designated member of care team.

- Staff time spent coordinating care with emergency department.

Assessment and treatment plan does not have to be comprehensive.

Services may be provided in any outpatient setting as long as the reporting professional has an ongoing relationship with the patient and clinical staff.

Services are provided face-to-face with patient or non-face-to-face.

SELECTING CODES USING TIME OR MDM

Code is selected using time only.

Time must be at least 20 minutes in a calendar month.

Do **NOT** report these codes:
- If time is less than 20 minutes in a calendar month.
- For time spent while the patient is inpatient or in observation care.

The time spent providing other services is **NOT** included in time used for to select this code.

(continued on next page)

PATIENTS
Patient has behavioral health condition, including substance use, that requires care management services.

PROVIDERS
The services are: • Provided by clinical staff. • Reported by a supervising physician or other qualified health care professional who is able to perform the E/M services required for an initial visit. Clinical staff must be available for face-to-face services with the patient. Clinical staff are **NOT** required to have qualifications that would permit them to separately report services (eg, psychotherapy), but if qualified, such services may be reported separately.

OTHER SERVICES
These services are **NOT** included in this code. Report separately if provided in the same month, but were distinct from 99484: • Psychiatric services (90785-90899). • Chronic care management services as long as services are separate (+99437, +99439, 99487, +99489, 99490, 99495, 99496). • Principal care management services (99424-99427). • Advance care planning (99497, +99498). • Counseling, risk factor reduction (99401).
Do **NOT** report 99484 in the same month as: • Psychiatric collaborative care management services (99492, 99493, +99494).
Do **NOT** report 99484 for the clinical staff time spent with a patient in inpatient/observation setting.

Psychiatric Collaborative Care Management Services

Psychiatric collaborative care management services are provided to a patient who requires a behavioral health care assessment to establish, implement, revise, or monitor a care plan, and/or provide a brief intervention.

The services are provided by a team: a treating physician, a behavioral health manager, and a psychiatric consultant). Codes are reported by the treating physician or other qualified health care professional. See page 66 for a list of services that the other providers may report.

Summary of Specific Criteria Used to Select Psychiatric Collaborative Care Management Codes

	Services	Medical Decision Making	Providers*	Time
99492	Initial service Psychiatric Collaborative Care Management		Clinical staff under supervision of physician or other QHP	First 70 minutes in first calendar month
99493	Subsequent service Psychiatric Collaborative Care Management		Clinical staff under supervision of physician or other QHP	First 60 minutes in subsequent month
+99494	Initial or subsequent service Psychiatric Collaborative Care Management		Clinical staff under supervision of physician or other QHP	Each additional 30 minutes in calendar month

*See next page for types of clinical staff who provide these services.
 Codes are reported by physician or other QHP.

Different Providers for Psychiatric Collaborative Care Management (99492, 99493, +99494)

Providers	Description	Services Provided
Qualified health care professionals	Treating physician or other qualified health care professional.	• Directs behavioral health care manager. • Oversees the patient's care. • Prescribes medications. • Treats medical conditions. • Makes referrals to specialty care when needed.
Behavioral health care manager	Clinical staff with a masters/doctoral-level education or specialized training in behavioral health.	• Provides face-to-face and non-face-to-face services to patient. • Works in consultation with a psychiatric consultant at least once a week (typically non-face-to-face). • Provides care management services. • Develops care plan. • Assesses patient needs. • Administers validated rating scales. • Provides brief interventions. • Maintains a registry.

Psychiatric consultant	Medical professional trained in psychiatry or behavioral health and qualified to prescribe the full range of medications.
	
	Provider has contracted directly with treating provider.
		• Typically communicates to the treating physician or other qualified health care professional through the behavioral health care manager.
		• Typically does not see the patient or prescribe medications.
		• Advises and makes recommendations, as needed, for psychiatric and other medical care including:
		  o Psychiatric and other medical differential diagnosis.
		  o Treatment strategies.
		  o Medication management (but usually does **NOT** prescribe medications).
		  o Management of medical complications associated with treatment of psychiatric disorders.
		  o Referring patient to specialty services.

Communication between these providers is as follows:
• Treating physician or other QHP directs the behavioral health care manager.
• Psychiatric consultant communicates through behavioral health care manager to the treating physician or other QHP.

Codes are reported by treating physician or other qualified healthcare professional.

Guidelines - Psychiatric Collaborative Care Management Services (99492, 99493, +99494)

GENERAL GUIDELINES

Each code includes:
- Activities of healthcare manager.
- Consultation between healthcare manager and psychiatric consultant.
- Direction of services by treating physician or other qualified health care professional.

Services include:
- Behavioral health care assessment.
- Establishing, implementing, revising, or monitoring a care plan.
- Providing brief interventions using evidence-based techniques such as:
  - Behavioral activation (using behaviors to influence emotional state).
  - Motivational interviewing.
  - Other focused treatment strategies.

These services are provided face-to-face with patient and non-face-to-face.

There are no separate codes for new and established patients.

There are separate codes for initial and subsequent care.

SELECTING CODES USING TIME OR MDM

These codes are selected using time only.

Time is calculating per month for each episode of care. An episode of care:
- <u>Begins</u> when treating physician or other qualified health care professional sends the patient to a behavioral health care manager.
- <u>Ends</u> when:
  - Targeted treatment goals are reached. This typically results in discontinuation of care management services and continuation of usual follow-up with treating physician or other qualified health care professional OR
  - Targeted treatment goals are **NOT** reached. Patient is referred to psychiatric care provider for ongoing treatment of behavioral health condition OR
  - Patient had no continued engagement with psychiatric collaborative care management services for six consecutive months (a break in the episode).

A new episode of care starts when patient is seen again after a break in care of 6 calendar months or more.

Do **NOT** use these codes if total time is less than 36 minutes.

Initial services code 99492 is reported for first 70 minutes in first calendar month of service. Time must be at least 36 minutes.
If more than 85 minutes of care are provided, report this code and code +99494. This add-on code can be reported in multiple units if appropriate.

Subsequent services code 99493 is reported for first 60 minutes in subsequent month of service, same episode of care.
Time must be at least 31 minutes.
If more than 75 minutes of care are provided, report this code and code +99494. This add-on code can be reported in multiple units if appropriate.

(continued on next page)

PATIENTS

Patient typically:
- Has behavioral health signs and/or symptoms OR
- Has a newly diagnosed behavioral health condition.
- Needs help in engaging in treatment.
- Has not responded to standard care delivered in a nonpsychiatric setting OR
- Requires further assessment and engagement prior to consideration of referral to a psychiatric care setting.

PROVIDERS

Services are <u>provided</u>:
- By behavioral health care manager.
- In consultation with psychiatric consultant.
- Under direction of treating physician or other qualified health care professional.

Codes are <u>reported</u> by:
- Treating physician or other qualified health care professional.

Sometimes a treating physician or other qualified health care professional <u>personally</u> performs some of the activities usually performed by a behavioral health manager.

In this case:
If the physician or other health care professional's activities are **NOT** being coded using another E/M code, then add their time to behavioral manager's time to select total time.

ENCOUNTERS

Initial Services

Initial services provided during a calendar month include:
- Outreach to and engagement in treatment of a patient directed by the treating provider.
- Initial assessment of the patient, including administration of validated rating scales, with development of an individualized treatment plan.
- Review by the psychiatric consultant with modifications of the plan if recommended.
- Entering patient in a registry and tracking patient follow-up and progress using the registry, with appropriate documentation.
- Providing brief interventions using evidence-based techniques such as behavioral activation, motivational interviewing, and other focused treatment strategies

If an initial service/new episode of care continues into additional calendar month(s), use subsequent service codes.

See section above on selecting code by time or MDM.

(continued on next page)

Guidelines - Psychiatric Collaborative Care Management Services (continued)

ENCOUNTERS (continued)

Subsequent Services

Subsequent services codes are reported when an episode of care continues into a new calendar month. Subsequent services include:

- Tracking patient follow-up and progress using the registry, with appropriate documentation.
- Participation in weekly caseload consultation with the psychiatric consultant.
- Ongoing collaboration with and coordination of the patient's mental health care with the treating providers.
- Additional review of progress and recommendations for changes in treatment, as indicated, including medications, based on recommendations provided by the psychiatric consultant.
- Monitoring of patient outcomes using calibrated rating scales.
- Relapse prevention planning with patients as they achieve remission of symptoms and/or other treatment goals and are prepared for discharge from active treatments.

See section on selecting code by time or MDM above

OTHER SERVICES

Qualified health care professionals may report these services in addition to collaborative management codes (99492, 99493, +99494):

- E/M services or other services separately during the same month.
- Psychiatric evaluation (90791, 90792).
- Psychotherapy (90832-90834, 90836-90840, 90846, 90847, 90849, 90853).
- Smoking and tobacco use counseling (99406-99407)
- Alcohol/substance abuse counseling (99408-99409).

Behavioral health care managers may report:

- Psychiatric evaluation (90791, 90792).
- Psychotherapy (90832-90834, 90836-90840, 90846, 90847, 90849, 90853).
- Smoking and tobacco use counseling (99406-99407)
- Alcohol/substance abuse counseling (99408, 99409).

These individuals may **NOT** report psychiatric collaborative care management codes (99492, 99493, +99494).

Psychiatric consultants may report:

- E/M services or other services separately during the same month.
- Psychiatric evaluation (90791, 90792).

These individuals may **NOT** report psychiatric collaborative care management codes (99492, 99493, +99494).

Time spent providing these services is **NOT** included in calculation of time for collaborative care management services.

Do **NOT** report 99492 and 99493 in the same calendar month for the same provider.

1. These codes can only be reported every 180 days:
   a. Cognitive assessment and care plan services
   b. General behavioral health integration care management
   c. Psychiatric collaborative care management

2. General behavioral health integration care management codes can **NOT** be reported during the same month as:
   a. Psychiatric collaborative care management
   b. Chronic management services
   c. Advance care planning
   d. Counseling, risk factor reduction

3. Psychiatric collaborative care management services include several different types of providers. Which of the following providers administer validated rating scales:
   a. Health care professionals
   b. Behavioral health care managers
   c. Psychiatric consultants

4. General behavioral health integration care management services are provided by:
   a. Clinical staff
   b. Physician or other qualified health care professional
   c. Advance practice nurse

5. For psychiatric collaborative care management, the psychiatric consultant communicates directly with:
   a. Treating physician or other QHP
   b. The behavioral health care manager
   c. The patient

6. The level of medical decision making for cognitive assessment and care plan services is:
   a. Straightforward
   b. Low
   c. Moderate or high
   d. No MDM is required

7. The cognitive assessment and care management services codes include a long list of included services. These codes can be reported:
   a. If six or more of these services are performed
   b. If any of these services are performed
   c. Only if all of these services are performed.

See Appendix B for quiz answers.

Chapter 15

CPT® Electronic and Telephone Services

Services can be provided on the telephone, online or using remote monitoring. These codes are summarized below.

Summary of Specific Criteria Used to Select Electronic and Telephone Codes

Codes		Individuals Involved	Time measured by -
99421-99423	Online Digital E/M services	Physician/qualified professional and established patient	Minutes
99441-99443	Telephone services	Physician/qualified professional and established patient	Minutes
99446-99452	Interprofessional telephone/internet/EHR Consultations	Consulting physician and treating/requesting physician	Minutes

Other E/M codes can be reported for services provided either face-to-face with patient or using telemedicine if appropriate. This is discussed in chapter 19 of this book.

Online Digital E/M Services

Online digital services are reported for an online encounter between a physician/qualified health care professional and a patient. These service may be provided through email or a patient portal.

Summary of Specific Criteria Used to Select Digital E/M Services

Codes		Individuals Involved	Face-to-Face or Non-Face-to-Face?	Time measured by -
99421-99423	Online Digital E/M services	Physician or other QHP and established patient	Non-face-to-face	Minutes

Specific Times Used To Select
Online Digital E/M Services (99421-99423)

Codes	Cumulative Time - Up to 7 Days
99421	5-10 minutes
99422	11-20 minutes
99423	21 or more minutes

Guidelines – Online Digital E/M Services (99421-99423)

GENERAL GUIDELINES

Report these codes for online encounters between a physician/qualified health care professional and a patient when:

- Online encounter was initiated by the patient or patient's guardian (eg, patient or guardian sends e-mail to provider).
- Problem is either a new or known condition.

Documentation of encounter must:

- Be on HIPAA-compliant platform (such as electronic health record, EHR portals, secure email, other digital applications).
- Be permanently stored (electronically or using a hard copy).

Other providers in the same group may provide the services listed below. These services are included in these codes:

- Evaluation, assessment, management of patient.
- Review of inquiry.
- Review of patient records or data.
- Interaction with clinical staff.
- Development of management plans including prescriptions or ordering tests.
- Subsequent communication with patient.
- All professional decision making, assessment, and subsequent management.

Services are provided non-face-to-face with patient/guardian.

There are no separate codes for new and established patients or initial or subsequent service.

(continued on next page)

Guidelines – Online Digital E/M Services (continued)

SELECTING CODES USING TIME OR MDM

Codes are selected by minutes during a 7 day period.

Provider/patient communication may not be synchronous (at the same time).

Time includes all professional decision making, assessment, and subsequent management by providers in the same group practice.

Report these codes in minutes spent with patient in a 7-day period.
- Time begins with:
  - Provider's initial, personal review of patient's inquiry OR
  - Provider's interaction with clinical staff focused on patient's problem.

- Time ends upon completion of 7 day period. Add together all time spent providing services during the 7 days.

Do **NOT** report time:
- For clinical staff as part of total time used to report these codes.
- Less than 5 minutes.

PATIENTS

Patient is established to the provider. Encounter may be initiated by patient or guardian.

PROVIDERS

Services provided by physician or qualified healthcare professional who may report an EM service.

OTHER SERVICES

A separate service may or may not be reported, depending on the circumstances.

Patient first had an E/M service, then initiates an online service:
- E/M service and online service are for unrelated problems. Report two codes: one for E/M service and one for online service.
- E/M service and online service are for the same or a related problem. Report only the E/M service. Do **NOT** report the online service separately.

Patient first had an online service, then had an E/M service:
- Online service and E/M service are for related or unrelated problem. Add together the time spent for each service. Report only an online services code. Do **NOT** report a separate E/M code.

(continued on next page)

OTHER SERVICES (continued)

Do **NOT** report these codes:
- If also reporting end-stage renal disease services (90951-90970).
- If also reporting E/M services on the same day (99202-99215, 99245).
- If services are related to a surgical procedure and are within postoperative period for the surgery.

Do **NOT** report these services if:
- Online service involves a <u>nonphysician</u> provider who may not report E/M services (such as speech therapists). See codes 98970-98972.
- Online communication was nonevaluative (giving test results, scheduling appointments, etc.).

Do **NOT** report these codes if also reporting these services for the <u>same communication</u>:
- INR monitoring services (93792, 93793).
- Patient education (98960-98962, 99071, 99078, 99080).
- Telephone services (98966-98968, 99441-99443).
- Online assessment, non-physician (98970-98972).
- Remote physiologic monitoring services (99091).
- Care plan oversight (99373-99380).
- Prolonged services on date other than face-to-face service (99358, +99359).
- Medical team conference (99366-99368).
- Online digital E/M services (99421-99423).
- Principal care management (99424-+99427).
- Chronic care management (+99437, +99439, 99487-99491).
- Transitional care management (99495, 99496).

A decision tree on the next page describes coding for online services.

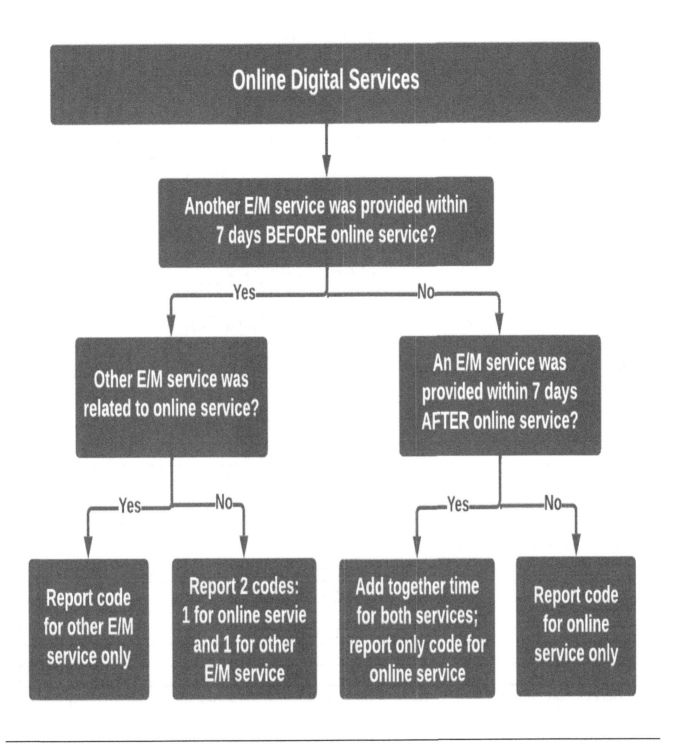

Online Digital Services

Another E/M service was provided within 7 days BEFORE online service?

— Yes → Other E/M service was related to online service?

- Yes → Report code for other E/M service only
- No → Report 2 codes: 1 for online servie and 1 for other E/M service

— No → An E/M service was provided within 7 days AFTER online service?

- Yes → Add together time for both services; report only code for online service
- No → Report code for online service only

The other E/M service may be face-to-face E/M visit or synchronous telemedicine visits using interactive audio and video telecommunication equipment, which are reported with modifier

173

Telephone Services

These codes are used to report an encounter between a physician/qualified professional and a patient using the telephone.

Summary of Specific Criteria Used to Select Digital E/M Services

Codes		Individuals Involved	Face-to-Face or Non-Face-to-Face?	Time measured by -
99441-99443	Telephone services	Physician or QHP and established patient	Non-face-to-face	Minutes

Specific Times Used to Select
Telephone Services Codes (99441-99443)

Code	Time
99441	5-10 minutes of medical discussion
99442	11-20 minutes of medical discussion
99443	21-30 minutes of medical discussion

Telephone Services (99441-99443)

GENERAL GUIDELINES
Report these codes for a telephone encounter between a physician/qualified health care professional and a patient.
Encounter is initiated by patient or patient's guardian (eg, patient or guardian calls provider).
These services are non-face-to-face.
There are no separate codes for new and established patients or initial or subsequent service.
SELECTING CODES USING TIME OR MDM
These codes are selected using time only.
PATIENTS
Patient is established to the provider.
PROVIDERS
Services are provided by a physician or other qualified health care professional who may report E/M services.
Do **NOT** report these codes if:
• Call involved a nonphysician provider who may **NOT** report E/M service (such as a speech therapist). See codes 98966-98968.

(continued on next page)

OTHER SERVICES

Do **NOT** report these codes if:
- Service was provided during the same month as chronic care management (99487, +99489).

Do **NOT** report these services if also reporting:
- Care plan oversight (99374, 99375, 99377-99380) for same call(s).
- INR monitoring services (93792, 93793).
- Online digital E/M services (99421-99423).

Do **NOT** report these services provided during the same service time as a telephone service:
- Transitional care management (99495, 99496).
- Principal care management (99424-99427).

Do **NOT** report these codes:
- If a decision is made to see the patient either within <u>24 hours</u> after the call or the next available urgent visit appointment.
- If a related E/M service was provided and reported within <u>7 days</u> before call.
- During postoperative period following a procedure.

A decision tree on the next page describes coding for telephone services.

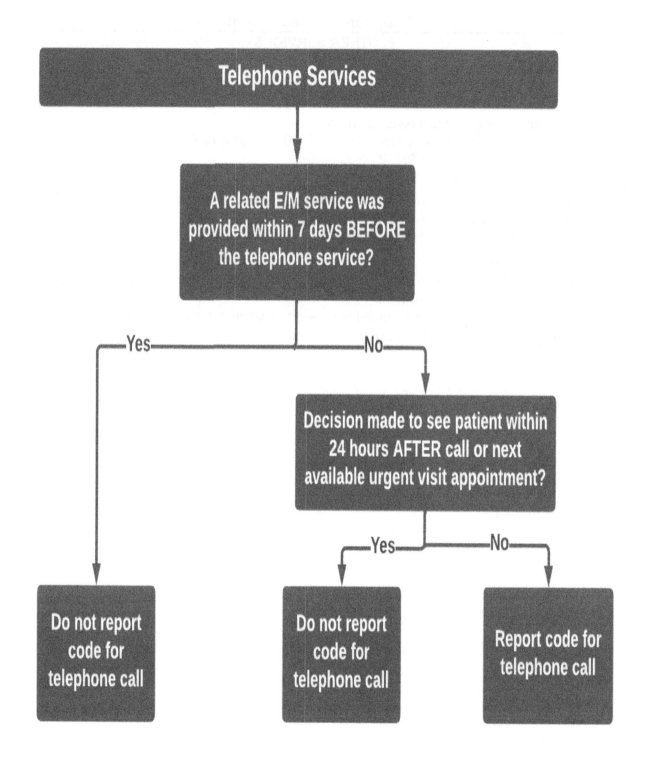

Telephone Services

A related E/M service was provided within 7 days BEFORE the telephone service?

Yes — Do not report code for telephone call

No — Decision made to see patient within 24 hours AFTER call or next available urgent visit appointment?

Yes — Do not report code for telephone call

No — Report code for telephone call

Interprofessional Telephone/Internet/EHR Consultation

Interprofessional telephone/internet/EHR consultations include an assessment and management of a patient.

Two providers are involved:
- The patient's treating (attending or primary) provider, who requests an opinion and/or advice from
- Another provider (the consultant), who has specific expertise in an area of concern for a specific patient.

Codes are selected by provider and time.

Summary of Specific Criteria Used to Select Interprofessional Telephone/ Internet/EHR Consultation Codes

Services		Individuals Involved	Face-to-Face or Non-Face-to-Face?	Time measured by -
99446-99452	Interprofessional telephone/ Internet/EHR Consultation	Two physicians or other QHP	Non-face-to-face	Minutes

For face-to-face consultation services, see codes 99242-99245, 99252-99255. These are discussed in chapter 4.

Different Providers for Interprofessional Telephone/Internet/EHR Consultations (99446-99452)

Code	Provider	Included Services	Minutes
99446	Consultative physician or other qualified healthcare professional	Consultation with verbal and written report sent to patient's treating/requesting physician or other qualified health care professional.	5-10 minutes of medical consultative discussion and review
99447	Consultative physician or other qualified healthcare professional	Consultation with verbal and written report sent to patient's treating/requesting physician or other qualified health care professional.	11-20 minutes of medical consultative discussion and review
99448	Consultative physician or other qualified healthcare professional	Consultation with verbal and written report sent to patient's treating/requesting physician or other qualified health care professional.	21-30 minutes of medical consultative discussion and review
99449	Consultative physician or other qualified healthcare professional	Consultation with verbal and written report sent to patient's treating/requesting physician or other qualified health care professional.	31 minutes or more of medical consultative discussion and review
99451	Consultative physician or other qualified healthcare professional	Consultation with written report only sent to patient's treating/requesting physician or other qualified health care professional.	5 minutes or more of medical consultative time
99452	Treating physician or other qualified healthcare professional	Consultation and referral services.	16-30 minutes Preparing for referral and/or communicating with consultant

Note: Codes 99446-99451 are reported by the consultant.

Code 99452 is reported by the treating/requesting provider.

Codes 99446-99449 include the consultant's verbal and written report sent to treating provider.

Code 99451 includes the consultant's written report only sent to treating provider.

Guidelines - Interprofessional Telephone/Internet/EHR Consultation (99446-99452)

GENERAL GUIDELINES

These codes are reported when a treating provider requests an opinion or advice from a consulting physician by telephone or other non-face-to-face communication.

Services include:
- Documentation of treating/requesting provider's written or verbal request for consultation, including reason for request.
- Review of medical records, lab and imaging studies, medications, pathology specimens.
- Verbal and/or written reports from consultant to treating physician.

Do **NOT** report these codes if:
- Consultation leads to a transfer of care.
- Only purpose of communication is transfer of care or other routine services.
- Consultation leads to face-to-face encounter with the patient <u>within</u> 14 days of services or next available appointment.
- Consultant has seen the patient face-to-face <u>within</u> the last 14 days.

The patient is not present during the consultation.

There are no separate codes for new or established patients or initial or subsequent service.

SELECTING CODES USING TIME OR MDM

These codes are selected by minutes in a 7-day period.
- Code for cumulative minutes over 7-day period. Report codes once for total time during a 7-day period.
- Report only one code for total time during the 7-day period, even if more than one communication occurred during the period.

Do **NOT** report these codes if consultation lasts less than 5 minutes.

PATIENTS

Patient may be either:
- A new patient or
- An established patient with a new problem or exacerbation of an existing problem

PROVIDERS

Service includes a communication between two physicians or other qualified health care professionals. The consulting physician has a specific specialty expertise that may assist the treating provider in the diagnosis and/or management of the patient's problem.

Codes reported by **consultant**:
- Codes 99446-99449 are reported when the consultant sends both a written and verbal report to the treating/requesting provider. Less than 50% of total time was devoted to data review and/or analysis rather than consultation.
- Code 99451 is reported when the consultant sends only a written report to the treating/ requesting provider. Use this code if total time is based on time spent in review and interprofessional-communication. More than 50% of total time was devoted to data review and/or analysis rather than consultation. This code can include as little as 5 minutes of consultative time.

(continued on next page)

179

PROVIDERS (continued)

Code reported by the **treating/requesting provider**: 99452.

Use this code if 16-30 minutes of total time was spent in preparing for the referral and/or communicating with the consultant during a service day.

Do NOT report this code more than once in a 14-day period.

OTHER SERVICES

Services **NOT** included in these codes. Report separately if appropriate:
- Face-to-face prolonged services codes +99417, +99418 can be reported by the treating/requesting provider if:
  - Time spent for the consultation exceeds 30 minutes beyond the time listed in the appropriate code AND
  - Patient is present (onsite) and accessible to treating/requesting physician or other qualified health care professional.

- Non-face-to-face prolonged services codes 99358, +99359 can be reported by the treating/requesting provider if:
  - Time spent for the consultation exceeds 30 minutes beyond the time listed in the appropriate code AND
  - Patient is not present.

Do **NOT** report these codes if:
- Reporting consultant communications with the patient and/or family. Use codes for nonphysician call (98966-98968), online digital services (99421-99423), or physician calls (99441-99443) instead.
- Consultant has seen the patient face-to-face within the last 14 days.
- Consultation leads to a transfer of care or other face-to-face service (eg, surgery, hospital visit, scheduled E/M visit) within the next 14 days or next available appointment date.

A decision tree on the next page describes coding for interprofessional telephone/internet/EHR consultations.

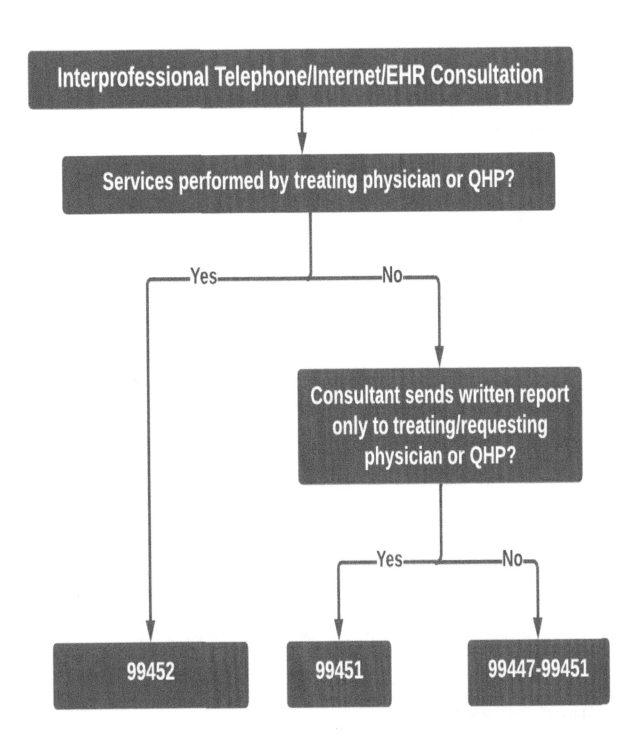

Interprofessional Telephone/Internet/EHR Consultation

Services performed by treating physician or QHP?

Yes / No

Consultant sends written report only to treating/requesting physician or QHP?

Yes / No

99452

99451

99447-99451

1. An E/M service was provided for a patient using an online digital method, in this case email. Five days later, a face-to-face visit for a related condition was provided. In this case:
   a. Add together the time for each service. Report only the online digital E/M service
   b. Report only the face-to-face visit
   c. Report both the online digital E/M service and the face-to-face visit

2. For telephone services codes, the call must be initiated by:
   a. The provider calling the patient
   b. The provider calling the patient's guardian
   c. The patient or guardian calling the provider

3. For interprofessional telephone/internet or EHR consultations, the services involve:
   a. The patient and a provider
   b. Two physicians or other qualified health care professionals
   c. Two patients

4. Code 99451 (interprofessional telephone/internet or EHR consultations), the services include:
   a. A consultation with verbal and written report
   b. A consultation with verbal report only
   c. A consultation with written report only
   d. Consultation and referral services only

5. When calculating time for an online digital service:
   a. Stop counting time 7 days after inquiry
   b. Start counting time when provider and patient begin online conversation
   c. Stop counting time 14 days following patient's initial contact.
   d. Start counting time 10 days after inquiry.

6. A telephone services code cannot be reported if:
   a. If the patient is seen 48 hours after the call (routine visit).
   b. If an E/M service related to the reason for the call occurs within 2 weeks of the call.
   c. If the patient is seen for the next available urgent visit appointment
   d. Six weeks following a minor procedure.

See Appendix B for quiz answers.

Chapter 16

CPT® Remote Physiologic Monitoring

These services include collection and use of digitally stored data. Codes are used to report equipment set-up, cost of the device, the actual monitoring, collection and interpretation of the data from the monitoring, and use of that data to treat or manage patient.

Summary of Criteria Used to Select Remote Physiologic Monitoring Services

Codes		Providers/Included Services	Minutes
99453	Digitally stored data services/ remote physiologic monitoring	Ordered by physician or other qualified healthcare professional. Set-up and patient education. Monitoring.	Each 30 days
99454	Remote monitoring of physio-logical parameters, device supply	Ordered by physician or other qualified healthcare professional. Includes device supply. Monitoring.	Each 30 days
99091	Collection and interpretation of physiologic data digitally stored and/or transmitted by the patient and/or caregiver to physician	Ordered by physician or other qualified healthcare professional. Collection and interpretation of data collected during monitoring.	Each 30 days
99457, +99458	Remote physiologic monitor-treatment management services	Clinical staff/physician/ qualified healthcare professional. Use of data collected and interpreted.	Minutes spent within a calendar month
99473	Self-measured blood pressure using a device validated for clinical accuracy	Provider performs education/ training and device calibration Patient measures their own blood pressure and reports the data to provider.	Not specified
99474	Self-measured blood pressure using a device validated for clinical accuracy; separate self-measurement of two readings one minute apart	Patient measures own blood pressure and reports data to provider. Provider collects data and communicates with patient concerning treatment plan.	Twice daily over a 30-day period; minimum of 12 readings

Separate codes are reported for:

- Preparing for and performance of remote monitoring services (99453, 99454, 99473, 99474).
- Collection and interpretation of data collected during the monitoring (99091).
- Use of data collected and interpreted to manage and treat patient (99457, +99458).

These services are described on the next few pages.

Preparing For and Performance of Remote Monitoring
(99453, 99454, 99473, 99474)

These codes are used for physiologic monitoring services. Different codes are used to report set-up and patient education, cost of the devices, and monitoring of physiologic parameter(s), eg, weight, blood pressure, pulse oximetry, respiratory flow rate.

Services are ordered by a physician or other qualified health care professional.

Summary of Specific Criteria Used to Select Digitally Stored Data Services/ Remote Physiologic Monitoring Codes

Codes		Time
99453	Remote monitoring of physiologic parameter(s) (eg, weight, blood pressure, pulse oximetry, respiratory flow rate), initial; set-up and patient education on use of equipment.	Report once per episode of care
99454	Remote monitoring of physiologic parameter(s) (eg, weight, blood pressure, pulse oximetry, respiratory flow rate), initial; device supply with daily recording(s) or programmed alert(s) transmission, each 30 days	Report each 30 days
Self-Measured (By Patient) Blood Pressure Monitoring		
99473	Self-measured blood pressure using a device validated for clinical accuracy; patient education/training and device calibration	Report once per device
99474	Self-measured blood pressure using a device validated for clinical accuracy; separate self-measurements of two readings one minute apart, twice daily over a 30-day period (minimum of 12 readings), collection of data reported by the physician and/or caregiver to the physician or other qualified healthcare professional, with report of average systolic and diastolic pressures and subsequent communication of a treatment plan to the patient	Report each 30 days

Code 99453 is reported once for the initial episode of care.

Code 99473 is reported once for each device.

Codes 99454 and 99474 are reported for the initial 30 days of monitoring or any subsequent 30 days during an episode of care.

Preparing For And Performance Of Remote Monitoring
(99453, 99454, 99473, 99474)

GENERAL GUIDELINES

These codes are reported for the preparatory services (patient education and device supply) and the actual remote monitoring.

Monitoring may be performed using a remote device (99453, 99454) or by patient for transmittal to providers (99473, 99474).

There are no separate codes for new or established patients or initial and subsequent services.

Codes are selected by time except for 99473.

For interpretation of the data obtained through the remote monitoring of physiologic parameter(s), see code 99091.

For use of data that has been collected to manage/treat the patient, see codes 99457 +99458.

Data Collected by Remote Device

Code 99453 – Patient education and set-up of device.
- Report this code for the set-up and patient education on use of device.
- Code is reported once for each episode of care. This:
  - Begins when remote monitoring physiologic service is initiated.
  - Ends when targeted treatment goals have been attained.

- Service must have been ordered by physician or other qualified health care professional.
- Service may be provided by clinical or non-clinical staff.

Device must have been:
- Validated for clinical accuracy.
- Defined as a medical device by U.S. Food and Drug Administration (FDA).

Code 99454 – Daily recording or programmed alert transmissions and device supply, each 30 days.
- Report this code for the cost of the device itself.
- Report this code for transmission of data.
- Service must have been ordered by physician or other qualified health care professional.

Device must have been:
- Validated for clinical accuracy.
- Defined as a medical device by U.S. Food and Drug Administration (FDA).

(continued on next page)

GENERAL GUIDELINES (continued)
Data Collected by Patient

Code 99473 – Report this code when the patient measures their own blood pressure and reports the measurements to the provider.

Code also includes:
- Patient education.
- Device calibration.
- Device validated for clinical accuracy.

Do **NOT** report this code more than once per device.

Code 99474 – Report this code when the patient measures their own blood pressure and reports the average systolic and diastolic pressures to the provider, over 30 day period.

Code also includes:
- 2 separate measurements performed 1 minute apart, twice daily over a 30-day period
- Minimum of 12 readings.
- Subsequent communication of a treatment plan to patient.

SELECTING CODES USING TIME OR MDM

Codes 99453, 99473 do not include a time component.
Codes 99454, 99474 are reported once every 30 days.

OTHER SERVICES

Do **NOT** report **99453**:
- More than once per device
- If monitoring is less than 16 days.
- When physiological monitoring services are included in time component of other codes (eg, code 95250 for continuous glucose monitoring, which requires a minimum of 72 hours of monitoring).
- For self-measured blood pressure monitoring. Use codes 99473, 99474 instead.
- For remote therapeutic monitoring. Use codes 98975-98977 instead.
- If reporting codes for more specific physiologic parameters (such as 93296, 94760).
- On the same day that patient receives an E/M service by the same provider.
- With remote multi-day complex uroflowmetry, patient education (0811T).

Do **NOT** report **99454**:
- If monitoring is less than 16 days.
- If reporting codes for more specific physiologic parameters (such as 93296, 94760).
- For self-measured blood pressure monitoring. Use codes 99473, 99474 instead.
- For remote therapeutic monitoring. Use codes 98975-98977 instead.
- With remote multi-day complex uroflowmetry, device supply (0812T).

(continued on next page)

OTHER SERVICES (continued)
Do **NOT** report **99473**:

Do **NOT** report **99473**:
- More than once per calendar month
- Chronic care management services (99490, 99491, +99437, +99439)
- Ambulatory blood pressure monitoring (93784, 93786, 93788, 93790)
- Collection and interpretation of data (99091)
- Principal care management services (99424, +99425, 99426, 99427)
- Remote physiologic monitoring (99453, 99454, 99457)
- Complex chronic care management (99487, +99389)
- Chronic care management (99490, 99491, +99437, +99439)

Do **NOT** report **99474**:
- On same day that patient receives another E/M service by the same provider.
- More than once per calendar month.
- Ambulatory blood pressure monitoring (93784, 93786, 93788, 93790)
- Collection and interpretation of data (99091)
- Principal care management services (99424, +99425, 99426, +99427)
- Remote physiologic monitoring (99453, 99454, 99457)
- Complex chronic care management services (99487, +99389)
- Chronic care management services (99490, 99491, +99437, +99439)

Collection and Interpretation of the Data (99091)

This code is reported for collection and interpretation of the data that was gathered during the remote monitoring.

Code	
99091	Collection and interpretation of the physiologic data.

Guidelines - Digitally Stored Data Services/Remote Physiologic Monitoring
COLLECTION AND INTERPRETATION of Remote Monitoring Data (99091)

GENERAL GUIDELINES
Code 99091 is reported for collection and interpretation of the physiologic data (eg, ECG, blood pressure, glucose monitoring). This code includes collection and interpretation of the physiologic data collected remotely, over a 30 day period. Report this code for physician or other QHP work to access data, review and interpretation of data, modify care plan as necessary and document work. Service are generally provided non-face-to-face with patient. For patient education, monitoring, and device supply, see codes 99453, 99454, 99473, 99474. For use of data that has been collected to manage/treat patient, see codes 99457, +99458.

SELECTING CODES USING TIME OR MDM
This code is reported for total time over a 30 day period. Time must be at least 30 minutes.

PATIENTS
Patient and/or caregiver may transmit data to physician or other qualified healthcare provider for interpretation.

OTHER SERVICES
Do **NOT** report this code if service occurs within 30 days when used to meet criteria for: • Care plan oversight services (99374, 99375, 99377-99380) • Physiologic monitoring (99457, +99458) Do **NOT** report this code: • More than once per 30 days. • On same day that patient receives another E/M service by the same provider. • If principal care management services were personally performed by provider during same service time (99424-+99427). • If a more specific codes exist for the services being provided (eg, 93227, 93272, 95250). • For transfer and interpretation of data from hospital or clinical laboratory computers.

Use of Data to Manage and Treat Patient (99457, +99458)

These codes are reported for use of data to manage and treat the patient under a specific treatment plan. This is the data that were collected by remote monitoring and interpreted (codes 99453, 99454, 99473, 99474, and 9901).

Specific Times Used for Remote Physiologic Monitoring Treatment Management Services (99457-99458)

Codes	
99457	First 20 minutes during a calendar month
+99458	Each additional 20 minutes during a calendar month

Guidelines – Remote Physiologic Monitoring Treatment Management Services (99457, +99458)

GENERAL GUIDELINES
Report these codes for provider's use of data that was collected by remote physiological monitoring to diagnose or treat patient under a specific treatment plan.
For patient education, monitoring and device supply, see codes 99453, 99454, 99473, 99474.
For interpretation of data, see code 99091.
SELECTING CODES USING TIME OR MDM
These codes are reported by minutes within a calendar month.
Time includes live, interactive communication (between provider and patient or caregiver).
The live communication does not need to represent the total time being reported. Total time can include
Code 99457 – First 20 minutes Code +99458 – Each additional 20 minutes
Report 99457 once regardless of number of physiologic monitoring modalities were performed in a month.
Report +99458 only if a full 20 minutes of additional care was provided. This code can be reported in multiple units when appropriate.
PROVIDERS
Service may be provided by physician, qualified healthcare professional, or clinical staff.

(continued on next page)

OTHER SERVICES

Services **NOT** included in these codes. Report separately if appropriate:
- Complex chronic care management services (99487, +99489).
- Behavioral health integration services (99484, 99493, +99494).
- Psychiatric collaborative care management services (99492, 99493, +99494).
- Chronic care management services (+99437, +99439, 99490, 99491).
- Transitional care management services (99495, 99496).

Do **NOT** count time spent providing these services in calculating time for physiologic monitoring codes.

Do **NOT** report these codes:
- Service time is less than 20 minutes.
- If reporting remote monitoring (93264, 99091).
- If more specific monitoring codes exist for the services being provided (such as cardiographic services 93227 or continuous glucose monitoring 99250).
- For set-up, education, and device supply. Use codes 99453-99474 instead.
- For remote therapeutic monitoring treatment management services. Use codes 98980, 98981 instead.

Do **NOT** count time spent on the following services towards time spent on monitoring on the same date:
- E/M services (99202-99205, 99211-99215).
- Home or residence services (99341, 99342, 99344, 99345, 99348-99350).
- Hospital inpatient/observation services (99221-99223, 99231-99233).
- Inpatient or observation consultations (99252-99255).
- Critical care services (99291, +99292).
- Time related to other reported services (93290, 93793).

A decision tree on the next page describes coding for remote physiologic monitoring services.

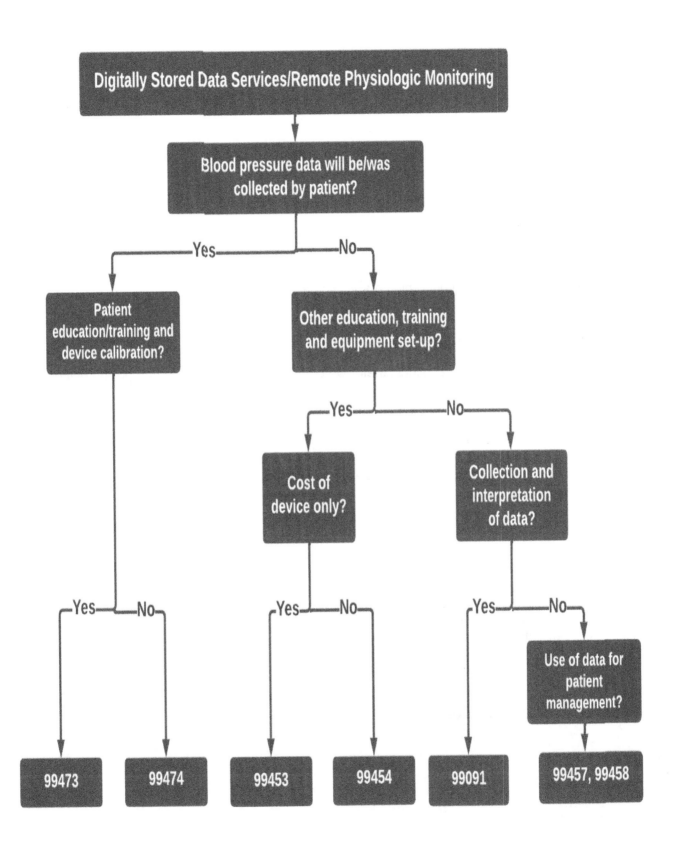

1. This code is reported once per episode of care:
   a. Code 99454
   b. Code 99453
   c. Code 99091
   d. Code 99474

2. For digitally stored data service/remote physiologic monitoring, the collection and interpretation of data are reported using code:
   a. 99453
   b. 99454
   c. 99091
   d. 99473

3. For use of the data collected digitally or through remote physiological monitoring for treatment decisions concerning a specific patient, use codes:
   a. 99453-99457
   b. 99457, +99458
   c. 99473-99474

4. Sometimes the patient collects their own blood pressure data. This is reported using code(s):
   a. 99453, 99454
   b. 99091
   c. 99473, 99474

5. Teaching a patient to use the device for monitoring is reported using code(s):
   a. 99453, 99473
   b. 99454, 99474
   c. 99091

6. Code 99457 is reported for services:
   a. Once per episode of care
   b. Once every 30 days
   c. First 20 minutes
   d. First 30 minutes

See Appendix B for quiz answers.

Chapter 17

Other CPT® Services

Not all E/M services fit neatly into one of categories listed in the previous chapters.

The codes described in this chapter do **NOT** include medically appropriate examination and history or medical decision making.

Some but not all of these codes include a time component.

Some but not all of these codes include face-to-face services.

Summary of Criteria Used to Select Codes for Other Services

Codes		Correct Code Determined by -	
		Direct face-to-face contact?	Time
99360	Standby services	No	√
99450	Basic life and/or disability evaluation services	Yes	
99455-99456	Work related/medical disability evaluation services	Yes	
99460-99463	Newborn care services	Yes	
99464-99465	Delivery/birthing room attendance and resuscitation services	Yes	
99497, +99498	Advance care planning	Yes	√
+99499	Pelvic examination	Yes	

Standby Services

This code is used to report non-face-to-face services standby services performed by physician or other qualified healthcare professional.

Summary of Criteria Used to Select Standby Services

Code	Time
99360 Standby Services	Each 30 minutes. Report code once for each full 30 minutes of standby provided. This code can be reported in multiple units when appropriate.

Guidelines – Standby Services (99360)

GENERAL GUIDELINES

Provider is asked to "stand by" (be available if needed) during services being provided by others, such as:
- Operative services
- Frozen section
- Cesarean/high risk delivery
- Monitoring EEG

Report these codes for services that:
- Are requested by another provider and
- Do **NOT** involve face-to-face encounter with patient.

SELECTING CODES USING TIME OR MDM

Codes are selected using time only.

Report code for each full 30 minutes of standby services.

Code can be reported in multiple units when appropriate.

Do **NOT** report these codes if:
- Total time is less than 30 minutes.

OTHER SERVICES

Services **NOT** included in this code. Report separately if appropriate:
- Initial hospital or birthing center care (99460).
- Delivery/birthing room resuscitation (99465).

Do **NOT** report this code if:
- After standing by, the providers performs face-to-face services with patient.
- The provider performs services to other patients while standing by.
- The provider proctors another individual while standing by.
- The period spent standing-by ends with the provider performing a procedure on the patient. (Exceptions: attendance at delivery [99460] and newborn services [99465]).
- Service was hospital mandated on-call services. See codes 99026, 99027.
- For initial hospital or birthing center care. See code 99464.

Newborn Care Services

These codes are used to report routine services provided to newborns, defined as infant aged birth through first 28 days.

Hospital/birthing center services are provided prior to initial discharge after birth.

Summary of Criteria Used to Select Newborn Care Codes

Codes	Location	Time
99460	Hospital or birthing center	Initial, per day, with overnight stay
99461	Not in hospital or birthing center	Initial, per day, with overnight stay
99462	Hospital	Subsequent, per day
99463	Hospital or birthing center	Admitted and discharged on the same date, per day

Guidelines – Newborn Care Services (99360-99463)

GENERAL GUIDELINES
Services provided include: • Documentation of maternal and/or fetal and newborn history. • Newborn physical examination. • Ordering of diagnostic tests and treatments. • Meetings with the family. • Documentation in medical record. Services are provided face-to-face with patient. Services may be in hospital or birthing center or outside these facilities. There are separate codes for initial and subsequent services. There are no separate codes for new and established patients.

SELECTING CODES USING TIME OR MDM
Codes are selected using time spent during initial/subsequent/same day admission and discharge and with/without overnight stay. No specific times are listed.

PATIENTS
Report these codes for services to newborns: • Described as "normal." * • Age birth through 28 days old. • Who have not been yet been discharged following birth.

*If patient has or develops an illness or condition that requires additional care, see codes for intensive, inpatient or critical care. Coding for this circumstance is described on the next page.

(continued on next page)

Guidelines – Newborn Care Services (continued)

ENCOUNTERS
Initial Encounter
For initial service, with overnight stay, use 99460 or 99461.
Subsequent Encounters
For subsequent service, use 99462.
Discharge Services
For same day admission and discharge, use 99463.
If patient is discharged after more than one day of newborn services, use hospital discharge services codes (99238, 99239).

MULTIPLE SETTINGS/SERVICES
Normal newborn later becomes ill and require additional services. Patient was not discharged. List two codes: one code for normal newborn care 99460-99463; and one codes for additional services. Use a modifier 25 on the additional services code.
Newborn was discharged to home, and then seen in follow-up in an office/outpatient setting by the same provider. List two codes: one code for newborn care; and one code for either office or other outpatient or preventive services codes as appropriate.

OTHER SERVICES
Services **NOT** included in these codes. Report separately if appropriate: • Delivery room attendance (99464). • Delivery room resuscitation (99465). • Routine procedures such as circumcision (54150).
Do **NOT** report these codes with: • Hospital inpatient services (99221-99223, 99231-99233). • Neonatal intensive care services (99477-99480). • Neonatal critical care services (99466, +99467, 99485, +99486).

Delivery/Birthing Room Attendance and Resuscitation Services

These services include provider's attendance during delivery and any resuscitation procedures provided at that time.

Summary of Criteria Used to Select Delivery/Birth Room Attendance and Resuscitation Codes

	Codes	Time
99464	Attendance at delivery when requested by delivering physician or other qualified health care professional. Initial stabilization of newborn.	No time designated
99465	Delivery/birthing room resuscitation Provision of positive pressure ventilation and/or chest compressions in presence of acute inadequate ventilation and/or cardiac output.	No time designated

Guidelines - Delivery/Birth Room Attendance and Resuscitation Services

GENERAL GUIDELINES
These services are reported for provider's attendance during a delivery and performance of procedures (initial stabilization or resuscitation).
SELECTING CODES USING TIME OR MDM
These codes are not selected using time or medical decision making.
OTHER SERVICES
Services **NOT** included in codes 99464, 99465. Report separately if appropriate: • Initial hospital inpatient/observation services (99221-99223). • Critical care (99291, 99468). • Initial newborn care services (99460). • Initial intensive care (99477). • Any procedures performed as a <u>necessary</u> part of resuscitation in addition to 99465. Examples are intubation, placing vascular lines.
Do **NOT** report: • Code 99465 with 99464. • Any procedures performed in the delivery/birthing room as a convenience before admission to the neonatal intensive care unit.

197

Disability Services

These codes include basic life and/or disability and work-related or medical disability evaluations. Different codes are used depending on patient's relationship to provider (99455-99456).

Summary of Criteria Used to Select Disability Services Codes

Codes	Provider
99450 Basic life and/or disability evaluation services	Not specified
99455 Work related or medical disability evaluation services	Treating physician
99456 Work related or medical disability evaluation services	Other than treating physician

Guidelines - Disability Services (99450, 99455, 99456)

GENERAL GUIDELINES

The codes list specific services that are provided:
- In office or other setting.
- To establish baseline information prior to issuing life or disability insurance certificates.

These services are provided face-to-face with patient.

There are no separate codes for new or established patient or initial and subsequent services.

Code 99450 (Basic life and/or disability evaluation services) includes:
- Measurement of height, weight, and blood pressure.
- Completion of a medical history following a standardized life insurance format.
- Collection of blood sample and/or urinalysis complying with "chain of custody" protocols.
- Completion of necessary documentation/certificate.

Codes 99455, 99456 (Work related or medical disability evaluation services) include:
- Completion of a medical history appropriate for the patient's condition.
- Performance of an examination appropriate for the patient's condition.
- Formulation of a diagnosis.
- Assessment of capabilities and stability and calculation of patient's impairment.
- Development of plan for future medical treatment.
- Completion of necessary documentation/certificates and report.

SELECTING CODES USING TIME OR MDM

These codes are not selected using either time or MDM.

PROVIDERS

For work related evaluation services:
- Report 99455 if services provided by physician who is <u>treating</u> the patient for injury/condition.
- Report 99456 if services provided by <u>another</u> physician (who is **NOT** treating the patient).

OTHER SERVICES

Services **NOT** included in these codes. Report separately if appropriate:
- Other E/M services provided on the same date.

Do **NOT** report these codes:
- With code for completion of workman's compensation forms (99080).
- If active management of problems was provided during the same encounter.

Advance Care Planning

These codes are used to report services to prepare an advance directive for the patient.
Examples of these directives are:
- Health care proxy
- Durable power of attorney for health care
- Living will
- Medical orders for life-sustaining treatment (MOLST)

Summary of Criteria Used to Select
Advance Care Planning Codes

Codes	Time
99497 Advance care planning	First 30 minutes
+99498 Advance care planning	Each additional 30 minutes

Guidelines – Advance Care Planning (99497, +99498)

GENERAL GUIDELINES

Codes are used to document patients decisions regarding their future medical treatment if they are unable to make these decisions themselves.

Services include:
- Face-to-face services between provider and family member or surrogate.
- Counseling, explanation, discussion and completion of forms for advance directives.

May or may not include completion of relevant legal forms.

These services involve a provider and family member or surrogate.

Code +99498 is an add-on code. It may be reported in multiple units when appropriate.

These services are provided face-to-face, via audio-only or using telemedicine services if appropriate.

There are no separate codes for new or established patients or initial or subsequent service.

SELECTING CODES USING TIME OR MDM

These codes are selected using time only.

Report code 99497 for first 30 minutes.

Report code +99498 for each additional 30 minutes. Can be listed in multiple units when appropriate.

OTHER SERVICES

Services **NOT** included in these codes. Report separately if appropriate:
- Office/other outpatient services (99202-99215).
- Hospital inpatient/observation care (99221-99223, 99231-99236, 99238-99239).
- Consultations (99242-99245, 99252-99255).
- Emergency department services (99281-99285).
- Nursing facility services (99304-99316).
- Home or residence services (99341-99350).
- Preventive medicine services (99381-99397).
- Transitional care management services (99495-99496).

Do **NOT** report these codes if active management of problem(s) is provided at same encounter.

Pelvic Examination

This is an add-on code used with other E/M codes listed below.

Guidelines – Pelvic Examination (+99459)

GENERAL GUIDELINES
This add-on code is used with other E/M codes to report that a pelvic examination was performed as part of the service.
SELECTING CODES USING TIME OR MDM
This code is not reported using either time or MDM.
OTHER SERVICES
Report this code with: • Office/other outpatient services (99202-99215). • Consultations (99242-99245, 99252-99255). • Preventive medicine care, patients 5 years of age or older (99383-99387, 99393-99397)

REVIEW – CHAPTER 17

1. A provider is asked to "stand by" for another provider, and then is called in the provide face-to-face services to that patient. In that case:
   a. Report the stand-by service only
   b. Report the face-to-face service only
   c. Report codes for both the stand-by and the face-to-face service.

2. Newborn care services are provided to patients 28 days or younger who:
   a. Are normal (no apparent abnormal conditions)
   b. Require critically ill services
   c. Require intensive care services

3. Disability services code 99450 includes all of these services EXCEPT:
   a. Completion of a medical history following a life insurance form.
   b. Collection of blood sample and/or urinalysis
   c. Measurement of height, weight, and blood pressure
   d. Completion of workman's compensation forms

4. Advance care planning services do **NOT** include:
   a. Health care proxy
   b. Living will
   c. Management of an active problem
   d. Counseling and completion of appropriate forms

See Appendix B for quiz answers.

Chapter 18

CPT® Modifiers and Symbols

The modifiers add important information to an E/M service to further define the service or the relationship of one service to another.

Summary of Modifiers Used with E/M Codes

Modifiers	Description
24	Indicates that two services were provided <u>during a postoperative period</u> by the same provider. The modifier is added to the E/M service to indicate that it was unrelated to the surgical service provided.
25	Indicates that two services were provided <u>on the same day</u> by the same physician or other qualified healthcare professional. One service was a procedure or other service. The modifier is added to the E/M service to indicate that it was a significant, separately identifiable service.
57	Indicates that an E/M service resulted in a <u>decision to perform</u> surgery. The modifier is added to the E/M service to indicate that the decision was made on the day before or day of the actual surgery.
93	Indicates that an E/M service was provided using synchronous telemedicine services via telephone or other real-time interactive <u>audio-only</u> telecommunications system.
95	Indicates that an E/M service has provided using synchronous telemedicine service using real-time interactive <u>audio or video</u>.

Modifiers are added to the end of CPT codes using a dash (eg, 99212-25).

Modifiers 24, 25, and 57 are used to pull an E/M service out of the global surgical package so that it can be reported and reimbursed separately. The global package is described on page 203.

Note that if these modifiers are not added to the E/M service, payers will assume that the service was part of the global surgical package and may not reimburse for the code separately.

Modifiers 24, 25 and 57 are often confused. When do you use each modifier?
- Modifier 24 – E/M service and procedure are <u>unrelated</u>. E/M service provided during the postoperative period for a procedure.
- Modifier 25 – E/M service and procedure are <u>related</u>. This modifier is generally used for minor procedures performed on at the same visit as the E/M service.
- Modifier 57 – E/M service and procedure are <u>related</u>. This modifier is generally used for more significant procedures. It may or may not be performed on the same date; it is performed during a global surgical package.

Modifiers 93 and 95 indicate services that may be reported using telemedicine if appropriate.

Examples of how these modifiers are used begin on page 206.

Symbols indicate that the services may be provided using telemedicine services and whether a code, guideline or introduction to a section was revised or added for the current year. Other symbols indicate that a code is an add-on code or out of numerical order.

Modifiers 93 and 95 and the star and announcement symbols go hand in hand to indicate services that may be reported using telemedicine if appropriate.

Summary of Symbols Used with E/M Codes

Symbols	Description
★	Indicates an E/M code that can be provided using telemedicine services. Used for interactive audio and video telecommunications system (modifier 95).
◀	Indicates an E/M service that can be provided using telemedicine services. Used for interactive audio-only telecommunications system (modifier 93).
▲	Indicates an E/M code that has been revised for the current year.
●	Indicates an E/M code that is new for the current year.
►◄	Indicates wording in a guideline or introduction to a section that is new or has been revised for the current year.
✚	Indicates that a code is an add-on code. It can only be used with another code.
#	Indicates that a code has been resequenced, meaning out of numerical order.

E/M Services and CPT Global Surgical Package

Service	Included in Global Package Services NOT reported separately	NOT included in Global Package Services may be reported separately
Pre-operative services	Routine services, such as: • Signing consent forms. • Pre-operative history and physical exam. • Prepping patient for surgery.	• E/M service that determined that the patient needed surgery. • Diagnostic tests and procedures. • Treatment of complications. • Treatment of conditions unrelated to the reason for the surgery.
Intra-operative services	Routine services such as: • Opening and closing the patient. • Local infiltration.	Other non-routine distinct services/ procedures.
Post-operative services	Routine services, such as: • Wound check. • Removal of sutures. • Discussion with patient about caring for wound. • Documentation of service. • Evaluation of patient in post-anesthesia recovery area.	• Treatment of complications. • Treatment of conditions unrelated to the reason for the surgery.

The above table describes the global surgical package according to CPT. Medicare defines the package somewhat differently.

Comparison – Medicare and CPT Global Surgical Packages Used with E/M Codes

Services Provided	Medicare Global Surgical Package	CPT Global Surgical Package
E/M service during which decision for surgery was made.	Not included. Use modifier 25 or 57.	Not included. Use modifier 25 or 57.
Related E/M services during postoperative/postprocedural period.	0, 10 or 90 days after the surgery.	No specific number of postoperative days.
Unrelated E/M service during postoperative period.	Not included. Use modifier 24.	Not included. Use modifier 24.

Description of Modifiers Used With E/M Services

Modifier 24 - Unrelated E/M service by same physician or other qualified health care professional during a postoperative period.

Sometimes an E/M service, provided during the postoperative period, is unrelated to the reason for the surgery.

For example: Patient seen in physician's office two days following a hysterectomy with complaint of a sore ankle. List an E/M service with a modifier 24.

Modifier 25 - Significant, separately identifiable E/M service by same physician or other qualified health care professional on the same day of a procedure or other service.

The service must be significant, meaning that it meets the requirements for a level of an E/M service. If it is not significant, a separate code is not reported.

The separate E/M service may be related to the symptoms or condition for which the original procedure and/or service was provided. This may be reported using two codes: one for the procedure or service; and one for the E/M service. Add a modifier 25 to the E/M service. Different diagnoses are not required for reporting of a procedure and an E/M services code on the same date.

For example:
- Patient seen in physician's office with a complaint of a sore throat. The provider performs an significant examination to evaluate the sore throat and then perform a biopsy of the back of their throat during this visit. Report two codes: a procedure code for the biopsy; and an E/M code for the services provided to evaluate the sore throat. Add a modifier 25 to the E/M service.
- Patient seen for a preventive E/M service. During the visit, the patient complains of a sore throat. The provider performs a significant examination and gives the patient a prescription. Report two codes: an E/M code for the preventive service; and an E/M code for the service to evaluate the sore throat. Add a modifier 25 to the second E/M service.
- Patient seen for a preventive E/M service. During the visit, the patient asks for a renewal of her prescription for birth control. She is having no adverse effects from using the medication. This is a minor service. Report only the preventive service. Do **NOT** report a separate E/M code for the prescription renewal.

Modifier 57 - Decision for surgery. The global surgical package does not include the E/M encounter when the physician decided that surgery was needed. This is reported using an E/M code. Add a modifier 57 to indicate that it is not part of the global surgical package. This applies if the E/M service is provided on the day of or day before the procedure. If the decision is made outside this timeframe (such as two weeks before the surgery), no modifier is necessary.

For example:
- Patient is seen for sore throat. After an examination, the physician decides that a bronchoscopy should be performed and schedules the procedure for later that day in an outpatient clinic. For this day, report two codes: an E/M code; and the appropriate surgical code. Add a modifier 57 to the E/M code.
- Patient is seen for planned bronchoscopy. Prior to the procedure, the physician explains the procedure and has the patient sign consent forms. These are routine services included in the procedure. Therefore, no separate E/M service is reported. Report only the bronchoscopy.

Modifier 93 - Synchronous telemedicine service rendered via telephone or other real-time interactive audio-only telecommunications system. The provider and the patient are in different locations and communicate using telephone or other real-time interactive audio-only communications system. The service must be significant enough to meet the requirements needed for a level of an E/M service.

The symbol ◀ goes hand-in-hand with modifier 93. The symbol, printed in front of a code, indicates that this E/M code can be provided either face-to-face with the patient or using telephone or other real-time interactive audio-only communication system. The service must be significant enough to meet the requirements needed for a level of an E/M service. If these services are provided using audio-only telemedicine, add modifier 93 to the E/M service. See chapter 15.

These E/M codes can be reported for services via audio-only telemedicine if appropriate:

Services	Codes
Behavioral change interventions, individual	99406-99409
Advance care planning	99497, +99498

Modifier 95 - Synchronous telemedicine service rendered via a real-time interactive audio and video telecommunications system. The provider and the patient are in different locations and communicate directly (at the same time) using an audio-video communications system. The service must be significant enough to meet the requirements needed for a level of an E/M service.

The symbol ★ goes hand-in-hand with modifier 95. The symbol, printed in front of a code number, indicates an E/M service that can be provided either face-to-face with patient or using audio-video telemedicine services. If these services are provided using telemedicine, add modifier 95 to the E/M code. See chapter 15.

These E/M codes can be reported for services via audio-video telemedicine if appropriate:

Services	Codes
Office or other outpatient services	99202-99205, 99211-99215
Subsequent hospital care	99231-99233
Consultations	99242-99245, 99252-99255
Subsequent nursing facility care	99307-99310
Behavioral change interventions, individual	99406-99409
Prolonged outpatient services on same date as other E/M service	+99417, + 99418
Transitional care management services	99495, 99496
Advance care planning	99497, +99498

1. The physician provided an E/M services during a post-operative period for a condition unrelated to the reason for the surgery. The code should:
    a. Use a modifier 23 on the E/M code
    b. Use a modifier 24 on the E/M code
    c. Use a modifier 25 on the E/M code
    d. Not use any modifier

2. The physician provided an unrelated E/M service on the same day as a surgery. In this case, the coder should:
    a. Use a modifier 24 on the E/M code
    b. Use a modifier 25 on the E/M code
    c. Use a modifier 24 on the surgical code
    d. Use a modifier 25 on the surgical code

3. Dr. White removed John's gallbladder. John is a Medicare patient. This procedure has a 90 day global package. He comes into the office 10 days after the surgery to see Dr. White because of a problem in his knee (an E/M service). The modifier used in this case is:
    a. 24
    b. 25
    c. 26
    d. 27

4. The physician provided an unrelated E/M service on the same day as a surgery.
    a. Use a modifier 57 on the E/M code
    b. Use a modifier 24 on the E/M code
    c. Use a modifier 25 on the E/M code
    d. Not use any modifier

5. The symbol ▲ means:
    a. This guideline has been revised this year.
    b. This code is out of numerical order.
    c. This code is new this year.
    d. This code was revised this year

6. The patient was brought in by her mother to the physician's office. The child was complaining of ear pain. The provider did an E/M service and determined that the patient had an ear infection. The provider scheduled an insertion of a ventilating tube next week (code 69436). The provider reports:
    a. An E/M code with a modifier 57 and code 69436.
    b. An E/M code without a modifier and code 69436.
    c. An E/M code only.
    d. Code 69436 only.

Chapter 19

Definition of CPT® Terms

Following are terms used in the Evaluation and Management section of CPT book.

Term	Definition
Acute illness or injury	Used in medical decision making. See chapter 1. Recent or new short-term problem. Condition may be described as uncomplicated or complicated, with systemic symptoms, or posing a threat to life or bodily function
Advance care planning	Services provided to assist patient in preparing an advance directive. See chapter 17. This document appoints an agent and/or records the patient's wishes concerning their future medical treatment if they are unable to make these decisions at that time.
Advanced practice nurse	Registered nurses with master's and/or doctorate degrees with advanced education and training beyond registered nurses. When working with physicians, these clinicians are considered as in the exact same specialty and subspecialty as the physician.
Analyzed	Used in medical decision making. The process of using data. See chapter 1.
Appropriate source	Used in medical decision making. See chapter 1. Includes professionals who are not health care providers but are involved in patient management. Examples are a lawyer, parole officer, case manager, or teacher.
Behavior change intervention/individual counseling	Services provided to individuals specific behavior that is often considered an illness in itself. See chapter 14. Examples are counseling concerning smoking and alcohol use.
Behavioral health care manager	Used in psychiatric collaborative care management services. See chapter 14. Clinical staff with a masters/doctoral-level education or specialized training in behavioral health.
Care plan oversight	Services in which a physician oversees complex and multidisciplinary modalities provided by different providers and used to treat a patient. Patient is not present during oversight services. See chapter 13.
Chronic illness	Used in medical decision making. See chapter 1. Problem with an expected duration of at least a year or until death of the patient. Condition may be described as stable or acutely worsening, poorly controlled or progressing. It may be severe and may or may not require hospitalization.

Term	Definition
Clinical staff	An individual who works under the supervision of a physician or other qualified health care professional. The staff members are allowed by law, regulation and facility policy to: • Perform or assist in providing a specific professional service but • Can **NOT** individually report that professional service, except when individual is: o Providing services reported by codes specifically designated as for clinical staff use (such as 99484, +99415) or o Reporting codes not requiring a physician (99211, 99281).
Comorbidities	A patient has two or more diseases or medical conditions at the same time. See chapter 1. These conditions may or may not be considered in selecting a level of service.
Concurrent care	A patient receives similar services provided on the same day by more than one provider. Each provider reports codes using the patient status (new or established) appropriate for the services that they <u>personally</u> performed.
Consultation	One physician (requesting physician) asks another (consulting physician) for their opinion, advice, or recommendations on how to treat a specific patient for a specific problem. See chapter 4. The consulting physician then sends back a report to the requesting physician with recommendations as to how this patient should be treated. May be provided in outpatient or inpatient setting. Medicare does not pay for consultation codes.
Counseling risk factor reduction	Type of preventive medicine visit. See chapter 11. Counseling provided either face-to-face or by telemedicine services to promote health and prevent illness or injury. The patient does not have a specific illness at the time of the counseling.
Covering or on-call services	One provider is on call for or covering for another provider. In this case, the other provider reports the appropriate new or established patient code as if the service had been performed by the first provider. For example, Provider A is covering for Provider B. Provider A sees Provider B's established patient. Provider A reports an established patient code even though Provider A has never seen the patient before.
Critical care	Physician directly delivers medical care to critically ill or injured patient. See chapter 6.
Digitally stored data services	See remote physiologic monitoring treatment management services.
Direction of emergency medical system, advanced life support	Codes used by providers to communicate with rescue personnel. See chapter 5. Two entities are involved: • A provider located in a hospital emergency or critical care department and • Ambulance or rescue personnel outside the hospital, in two-way voice communication with the provider.
Disability services	Codes for basic life and/or disability and work-related or medical disability evaluations. See chapter 17.

Term	Definition
Discharge service	Services provided on the day that the patient is discharged from observation or inpatient care or a nursing facility. May be on same day as the admission or after the initial day.
Discussion	Used in medical decision making. See chapter 1. Discussion requires a direct, interactive exchange with another individual. May be asynchronous (communication using electronic means or other messaging, but not at the same moment). May **NOT** be through intermediaries (eg, information relayed through clinical staff or trainees).
Drug therapy	Used in medical decision making. See chapter 1. Monitoring a drug that has the potential to cause serious morbidity or death. Includes assessment of adverse effects of the drug over the long or short term.
Elective surgery	Used in medical decision making. See chapter 1. Procedure typically was planned in advance (eg, scheduled for days or weeks later).
Emergent surgery	Used in medical decision making. See chapter 1. Procedure typically performed immediately or with minimal delay to allow for patient stabilization.
Emergency department care	Services in a hospital area designed for unplanned care for patients who need immediate attention. Area is open 24 hours a day. See chapter 5.
Established patient	Person has received professional services within the last 3 years either from: • A physician in this group practice OR • Another physician in the same group practice of the exact same specialty and subspecialty. Example: Two maternal-fetal medicine specialists are the same group practice. Patient seen by Specialist A and then by Specialist B. The patient is considered established for Specialist B even if the specialist has never seen the patient before.
Evaluation and management codes (E/M)	Used to report non-surgical services. The codes are used to report the work the provider does to evaluate/diagnose a patient's condition.
External	Used in medical decision making. See chapter 1. Tests, records or communications from provider either: • Outside of primary provider's group, or • In same group but with providers with different specialty. May also be a facility or home health agency.
Face-to-face service	Services in which patient and provider are in the same room, seeing each other face-to-face. Also referred to as "with direct patient contact."
General behavioral health integration care management	Services provided by clinical staff to a patient with a behavioral health condition that requires case management. See chapter 14.

Term	Definition
Health care professionals	Individual provided psychiatric collaborative care management services. See chapter 14. Treating physician or other qualified health care professional directs behavioral health care manager and oversees patient's care. See also qualified health care professionals.
High severity	Used in medical decision making. See chapter 1. A problem where the: • Risk of morbidity without treatment is high to extreme • Risk of mortality without treatment is moderate to high or • Probability of severe, prolonged functional impairment is high.
Hospital outpatient clinic	Outpatient area within a facility. See chapter 2. Patient has not been admitted as inpatient.
Independent historian	An individual (parent, guardian, surrogate, spouse, witness) who provides a patient's history in addition to the history provided by the patient. See chapter 1.
Independent interpretation	Provider interprets a test performed by this physician or another individual. An interpretation is not the same as review of results. There must be a CPT code for the test and an interpretation is customary for this test.
Initial service	Services provided to a patient on the day the patient was admitted to hospital or observation care.
Inpatient services	Patient has been admitted to the hospital as an inpatient. See chapter 3.
Insignificant or trivial problem	See modifier 25 in chapter 18. A problem that does not require the provider to perform additional work beyond the usual preventive medicine services. No additional E/M code is reported.
Intensive care services	Used to report services to a child who is not critically ill but requires intensive observation, frequent interventions, and other intensive care services due to his or her low birth weight. See chapter 7.
Interprofessional telephone/Internet/ EHR consultations	Codes used to report a communication between two providers via tele-phone, the internet or other electronic means. The patient is not present. See chapter 15.
Low severity	Used in medical decision making. See chapter 1. A problem for which the patient's risk of morbidity without treatment is low.
Minimal problem	Used in medical decision making. See chapter 1. Problem that may not require the presence of the physician or other qualified health care professional. Service is supervised by physician or other qualified health care professional. See codes 99211, 99281.
Moderate severity	Used in medical decision making. See chapter 1. A problem for which the risk of mortality without treatment is moderate. Also used for patient conditions with uncertain prognosis or increased probability of prolonged functional impairment.
Modifiers	Two digit numbers that are added to the end of a CPT code. See chapter 18. With E/M codes, modifiers may be used to indicate that an E/M service is not included in the surgical global package, another E/M service or that the service can be provided using telemedicine.

Term	Definition
Morbidity	Used in medical decision making. See chapter 1. A state of illness or functional impairment that is expected to be of substantial duration.
Mortality	Used in medical decision making. See chapter 1. Risk of patient's death even with treatment.
New patient	Person has: • Never received professional services from any physician in this group practice OR • Was last been seen by this physician more than 3 years ago OR • Was seen within 3 years by another physician in this practice who has a different specialty. Example: obstetrician and maternal-fetal medicine specialist in same group practice. Each provider may report a new patient code.
Newborn services	Services provided to newborn before their discharge. A newborn is aged birth through first 28 days. See chapter 17.
Non-face-to-face service	Services in which patient and provider are not in the same room, not seeing each other face to face. Includes communicating via telephone, video or computer messaging. Also referred to as "without direct patient contact."
Nursing facility	Services provided in nursing facility, skilled nursing facility, intermediate care facility, long-term care facility, or psychiatric residential treatment facility. See chapter 8.
Observation	Care provided in a specific area of the hospital designated as observation department or other area of a hospital. Includes initiation of observation status, supervision of care plan and performance of periodic reassessments. See chapter 3.
On-call services	See covering services.
Online digital E/M services	Codes used to report an online communication between a provider and a patient. Examples are communication through email or a patient portal. See chapter 15.
Outpatient services	A patient who has **NOT** been formally admitted to a facility as an inpatient. Includes physician's office and hospital clinic. See chapter 2. The broad definition of outpatient includes individuals in settings such as emergency department or observation care, or other types of services, such as outpatient consultation. However, these settings and types of services have their own set of codes in CPT and are discussed in separate chapters in this book.
Per day services	Some categories of codes (such as hospital inpatient and observation care services and nursing facility services) are reported "per day." If multiple visits by one provider occur over the course of a single calendar date in the same setting, a single code is reported. These codes may be selected using either MDM or total time spent with the patient on a single day. • **Code selected using MDM**: Use the aggregated (combined) MDM elements over the course of the calendar date. • **Code selected using time**: Sum the time over the course of the day using the guidelines for reporting time.

Term	Definition
Physician or other qualified healthcare professional (QHP)	See Qualified healthcare professional.
Preventive medicine services	Patient is not sick but is being seen for services such as annual check-ups or well-baby visits. See chapter 11.
Principal care management services	Services provided to a patient with a single, complex chronic condition expected to last at least 3 months. See chapter 13. The encounter focuses on the patient's medical and/or psychological needs related to the condition.
Problem	Used in medical decision making. See chapter 1. A disease, condition, illness, injury, symptom, sign, finding, complaint, or other matter addressed at the encounter. A diagnosis may or may not be established at the time of the encounter.
Problem addressed	Used in medical decision making. See chapter 1. A problem that is evaluated or treated by the physician or other qualified health care professional reporting the service. Includes consideration of possible further testing or treatment that may ultimately not be performed after a risk/benefit analysis or due to patient/ parent/ guardian/surrogate choice.
Professional services	Face-to-face services provided by physicians and other qualified health care professionals who may report E/M services. See definitions of new and established patients.
Psychiatric consultant	Individual providing psychiatric collaborative care management services. See chapter 14. A medical professional trained in psychiatry or behavioral health and qualified to prescribe the full range of medications.
Qualified health care professional (QHP)	An individual who is qualified by education, training, licensure/regulation (when applicable), and facility privileging (when applicable). This individual: • Performs a professional service within their scope of practice and • Independently reports that professional service. Examples of QHP are: • Physician • Certified Nurse Mid-Wife (CNM) • Certified Registered Nurse Anesthetist (CRNA) • Clinical Nurse Specialist (CNS) • Clinical Social Worker (CSW) • Nurse Practitioner (NP) • Physician Assistant (PA) • Physical Therapist (PT) Sometimes a physician or other QHP is abbreviated in this book as "provider" to include physicians and QHP.
Remote physiologic monitoring treatment management services	Services provided by clinical staff/physician/other qualified health care professional. See chapter 16. Codes used for equipment set-up, monitoring devices, the actual monitoring, collection and interpretation of the data, and use of data to treat/manage patient.

Term	Definition
Risk	Used in medical decision making. See chapter 1. The probability and/or consequences of an event (morbidity, mortality, or adverse effect of treatment). The risk from the patient's condition is different than the risk of the treatment/management of the condition.
Self-limited or minor problem	Used in medical decision making. See chapter 1. Problem that runs a definite and prescribed course, is transient in nature, and is not likely to permanently alter health status.
Shared visit	See split or shared visits
Significant problem	See modifier 25. See chapter 18. A problem that requires the physician to perform additional work, including the components of an E/M code.
Social determinants of health	Used in medical decision making. See chapter 1. Economic and social conditions that influence the health of people and communities. Examples are: food insecurity, living alone, homelessness.

Split or shared visits	Sometimes two providers work together as a team to provide care for a patient during a single E/M service. Only one provider may report the service.
	
	Codes may be selected using either time or medical decision making (MDM):
	• **Total time on date of the encounter**: The service is reported by the provider who spent the majority of the face-to-face or non-face-to-face time with the patient.
	
	• **MDM level:** the service is reported by the provider who performed the substantive part of the MDM.
	  o The provider made or approved the management plan and taken responsibility for that plan with its inherent risks arising from patient management. This covers these elements of MDM: number and complexity of problem addressed and risk of complications and/or morbidity or mortality.
	  o The level of MDM may also include amount and/or complexity of data to be reviewed. In order to count this element, the provider does not have to personally assess an independent historian's narrative and order or review of tests or documents, but must personally interpret tests and discuss the management plan.

Standby Services	Provider stands by until or if needed to perform services: during operations; for frozen sections; for cesarean or high risk deliveries or for monitoring EEG. See chapter 17. Provider does not have any direct contact (face-to-face contact) with patient.
Subsequent service	Services provided on day after initial visit. May be reported several times if patient is an inpatient for three or more days.

Term	Definition
Synchronous	Communication at the same time, such as a conversation using a telephone. See chapter 15. A nonsynchronous conversation would be when one individual sends a message to the other; the other responds minutes or hours later. See chapter 15.
Telemedicine	Services in which patient and provider are not in the same room but are communicating using online conferencing or audio tools. See chapter 15. Services may be via audio only or audio-video. Synchronous service must meet the requirements of the same service if the services had been provided during a face-to-face encounter. The benefits of performing the service must be documented. See chapter 15.
Telephone services	Codes used to report a telephone call between a provider and a patient. Call is initiated by patient, not the provider. See chapter 15.
Test	Used in medical decision making. See chapter 1. Includes collection of imaging, laboratory, psychometric or physiologic data.
Transfer of care	Sometimes one provider is managing some or all of a patient's problem but then transfers this responsibility to another provider. The first provider may still care for other conditions. The second provider must: • Explicitly agree to accept responsibility for patient and • Beginning with the initial encounter, must not provide consultative services. Each provider reports codes with specific services/appropriate patient status for services that they personally performed.
Transitional care management services	Services for any needed coordination of care performed by multiple disciplines and community service agencies when a patient is being transferred from one facility to another location. See chapter 12.
Undiagnosed new problem with uncertain prognosis	Used in medical decision making. See chapter 1. Problem documented using a differential diagnosis (eg, condition A vs condition B). Condition is likely to result in a high risk of morbidity without treatment.
Unique source	Used in medical decision making. See chapter 1. Data from a physician or qualified health care professional in a distinct group or different specialty or subspeciality, or a unique entity other than the provider who is providing the interpretation.
With direct patient contact	Provider and patient are in the same location, communicating face-to-face.
Without direct patient contact	Provider and patient are not communicating face-to-face.

1. Dr. A is on-call for Dr. B. Dr. A sees an established patient of Dr. B. Dr. A has never seen this patient before. Dr. A reports the visit as:
   a. Subsequent service
   b. New patient
   c. Initial service
   d. Established patient

2. A new patient is defined as a patient who has not seen the physician or any physician of the same specialty in the same group practice:
   a. Within the last year
   b. Within the last 2 years
   c. Within the last 3 years
   d. Within the last 4 years

3. A patient has been seeing Dr. A, a dermatologist in a multispecialty practice, for years. The patient then sees Dr. B, an orthopedist, who belongs to the same practice. His last visit with Dr. A was one year ago. For the visit with Dr. B, the patient is considered a:
   a. New patient
   b. Established patient
   c. Initial patient
   d. Subsequent patient

4. Physician A asks Physician B to take over care for a specific problem for this patient. This is referred to as a:
   a. Transitional care management
   b. Transfer of care
   c. Shared visit
   d. Concurrent service

5. A qualified healthcare professional (QHP) may be:
   a. Certified nurse midwife
   b. Nurse practitioner
   c. Physician assistant
   d. Physician
   e. All of the above

6. Codes that are reported per day can be selected:
   a. Using time only
   b. Using MDM only
   c. Using cumulative time or MDM elements for the whole date

Appendix A

Selecting a CPT® E/M Code Using Time and Medical Decision Making

The form on the following page can be used to help select the correct E/M code. This form can be used for codes that are determined by medical decision making and/or time. These are:

- Office and other outpatient services
- Hospital inpatient and observation services
- Consultations
- Nursing facilities
- Home or residence

The correct code is determined by answers to these questions:

1. Is patient new or established patient?

2. Is this an initial or subsequent encounter?

3. Where was the service provided?

4. Was this a consultation?

5. Which set of codes should be used?

6. What time was documented?

7. What level of MDM was documented?

8. What code would be selected using time and MDM?

9. Which code is reported?

Not all of these questions will apply to every encounter.

For codes that are selected using time only, MDM only, or other criteria, see appropriate chapter.

For more complicated cases, including multiple settings or multiple providers, see appropriate chapter.

The form is on the following page. Readers may duplicate this form as needed.

Examples of how to use the form are found on page 219.

Selecting an E/M Code
Using Time or Medical Decision Making

1. Is patient new or established?   _____

2. Is this an initial or subsequent encounter?   _____

3. Where was the service provided?   _____

4. Was this a consultation?*   _____

5. Which set of codes should be used?   _____

6. What time was documented?   _____

7. What level of MDM is documented?   _____
   Based on elements a), b) and c) below

   a) Number/complexity of problems   _____

   b) Amount/complexity of data   _____

   c) Risk of morbidity/mortality   _____

(To use a specific level of MDM, 2 of the 3 elements above must be met or exceeded. If each component is a different level, use the one in the middle.)

8. Turn to appropriate set of codes in the CPT book based on question 5.
   From these codes, select the code that matches the time (question 6) and MDM (question 7) documented for this encounter.

                                                       CPT Code

   Code based on TIME   _____

   Code based on MDM   _____

9. Which code is reported?   _____

   (Use whichever code from question 8 is higher)

*For consultations in an inpatient, observation, nursing facility or partial hospital setting, use inpatient consultation codes.
For consultations in an office, other outpatient, home or residence setting, use outpatient consultation codes.

Example 1: New patient seen in physician's office for 30 minutes. The physician documents straightforward level of number/complexity of problems, straightforward level of amount/ complexity of data, and low level of risk MDM.

Selecting an E/M Code Using Time or Medical Decision Making

1. Is patient new or established? _New_

2. Is this an initial or subsequent encounter? _Initial_

3. Where was the service provided? _Physician's office_

4. Was this a consultation?* _No_

5. Which set of codes should be used? _99202-99205_

6. What time was documented? _30 minutes_

7. What level of MDM is documented?
   Based on elements a), b) and c) below _Straightforward_

   a) Number/complexity of problems _Straightforward_

   b) Amount/complexity of data _Straightforward_

   c) Risk of morbidity/mortality _Low_

(To use a specific level of MDM, 2 of the 3 elements above must be met or exceeded. If each component is a different level, use the one in the middle.)

8. Turn to appropriate set of codes in the CPT book based on question 5.
   From these codes, select the code that matches the time (question 6) and MDM (question 7) documented for this encounter.

	CPT Code
Code based on TIME	_99203_
Code based on MDM	_99202_
9. Which code is reported?	_99203_

(Use whichever code from question 8 is higher)

*For consultations in an inpatient, observation, nursing facility or partial hospital setting, use inpatient consultation codes.

For consultations in an office, other outpatient, home or residence setting, use outpatient consultation codes.

Example 2: Patient seen for consultation. She was admitted yesterday but has not seen this provider before (or anyone from the admitting provider's practice). The consultation lasts 40 minutes. The physician documents low level of number/complexity of problems, moderate level of amount/complexity of data, and high level of risk MDM.

Selecting an E/M Code Using Time or Medical Decision Making

1. Is patient new or established?   *N/A*

2. Is this a initial or subsequent encounter?   *N/A*

3. Where was the service provided?   *Facility*

4. Was this a consultation?*   *Yes*

5. Which set of codes should be used?   *99252-99255*

6. What time was documented?   *40 minutes*

7. What level of MDM is documented?
    Based on elements a), b) and c) below   *Moderate*

    a) Number/complexity of problems   *Low*

    b) Amount/complexity of data   *Moderate*

    c) Risk of morbidity/mortality   *High*

(To use a specific level of MDM, 2 of the 3 elements above must be met or exceeded. If each component is a different level, use the one in the middle.)

8. Turn to appropriate set of codes in the CPT book based on question 5. From these codes, select the code that matches the time (question 6) and MDM (question 7) documented for this encounter.

	CPT Code
Code based on TIME	*99252*
Code based on MDM	*99254*

9. Which code is reported?   *99254*

    (Use whichever code from question 8 is higher)

*For consultations in an inpatient, observation, nursing facility or partial hospital setting, use inpatient consultation codes.

For consultations in an office, other outpatient, home or residence setting, use outpatient consultation codes.

Appendix B

Review Quiz Answers

REVIEW – CHAPTER 1

Selecting a CPT® Evaluation and Management Code

1. Medical decision making (MDM) is based on the:
    a. Number of diagnoses the physician must consider
    b. Patient's risk of morbidity
    c. Amount of data the physician must evaluate
    d. All of these elements are part of the MDM. √

2. An appropriate examination and history is determined by:
    a. Centers for Medicare and Medicaid Services
    b. The physician providing the service √
    c. The medical coder
    d. Definition in the E/M guidelines

3. A provider documents two self-limited or minor problems. For the number and complexity of problems addressed component of MDM, this is:
    a. Straightforward level
    b. Low level √
    c. Moderate level
    d. High level

4. A patient's condition is improving (meeting treatment goals), but not yet resolved. This condition is considered:
    a. Complicated
    b. Acute
    c. Chronic
    d. Stable √
    e. Unstable

5. For the high level of amount and/or complexity of data to be reviewed and analyzed, use of an independent historian is part of:
    a. Category 1 √
    b. Category 2
    c. Category 3

6. An example of high risk of morbidity is:
    a. Decision for elective major surgery without identified patient or procedure risk factors
    b. Treatment significantly limited by social determinants of health
    c. Prescription drug management
    d. Drug therapy requiring intensive monitoring for toxicity √

7. A provider documents this MDM: number/complexity of problems addressed – low; amount/complexity of data reviewed and analyzed – moderate; risks of management – low. The MDM for this patient is:
   a. Straightforward
   b. Low √
   c. Moderate
   d. High

8. Do not count total time for:
   a. Face-to-face encounters with the provider and patient and/or family/caregiver
   b. Non-face-to-face time spent with the patient and/or family/caregiver on date of encounter
   c. Time spent by the provider traveling to patient's location √
   d. Ordering medications for the patient

REVIEW – CHAPTER 2
CPT Office or Other Outpatient Services

1. A physician sees a new patient who had received a severe beating in a mugging. He treats the wounds and counsels the patient, who is quite traumatized by the event. The physician documents straightforward medical decision making. Code 99202 has a time threshold of 15 minutes. However, the physician spent a total of 30 minutes (code 99203) with this patient because of the exam and counseling. The coder reports:
    a. Code 99202
    b. Code 99203 √
    c. Code 99204
    d. Code 99205

2. A physician sees an established patient. She provides moderate level of medical decision making. The encounter lasts 25 minutes. The coder reports:
    a. Code 99211
    b. Code 99212
    c. Code 99213
    d. Code 99214 √

3. Which of these elements are NOT used to select an outpatient code:
    a. Examination and history √
    b. Time
    c. Medical decision making
    d. New or established patient

Hospital Inpatient and Observation Care Services

1. Which of these hospital/observation care codes do NOT include medical decision making?
   a. 99222
   b. 99234
   c. 99236
   d. 99238 √

2. An initial service is reported for hospital/observation care codes is defined as:
   a. When the patient has not received any previous professional services from the provider during this stay √
   b. When the patient has not received any professional services from the provider during the last 3 years
   c. When the patient is being discharged from inpatient/observation care

3. A discharge code is reported when the patient was admitted on:
   a. On the same date √
   b. On a different date

4. The provider saw the patient for 2 hours in the morning and 3 hours in the afternoon on the same day The time component is:
   a. 2 hours
   b. 3 hours
   c. 5 hours √
   d. Reported with two separate codes, one for 2 hours in the morning and another for 3 hours in the afternoon.

5. The provider saw the patient at 11 pm on Tuesday and stayed with the patient until 2 am the next day. The time component is:
   a. 1 hour
   b. 2 hours
   c. 3 hours √
   d. Reported with two separate codes, one for 11-12 pm and another for 12-2 am.

6. The coder is reporting a code for the second day that the patient is in observation care. The coder selected a code for:
   a. Initial service
   b. Subsequent service √
   c. Discharge service
   d. Prolonged service

7. Provider performed a consultation in their office. Following the consultation, this same provider admitted the patient to the hospital. In this case, the coder selected:
   a. A code of the outpatient consultation and a code for the an initial inpatient code.
   b. A code for the outpatient consultation and a code for a subsequent inpatient service √
   c. Only a code for the outpatient consultation.
   d. Only a code for the initial hospital admission.

8. Dr. Smith performed a consultation in the emergency department. The patient was then admitted by Dr. Jones. After the admission, Dr. Smith saw the patient again in consultation. For Dr. Smith, the coder selected:
    a. A code for the consultation and another code for initial hospital care.
    b. A code for the consultation and another code for subsequent hospital care √
    c. A code for the consultation only.
    d. A code for the initial hospital care only.

9. Provider admits patient to the hospital at 9:00 am on Tuesday. The patient is hen discharged by the same provider at 3:00 on the same date. This is reported using:
    a. Same day admission and discharge codes
    b. Initial service codes√
    c. Discharge service codes
    d. Initial and discharge service codes

225

REVIEW – CHAPTER 4
Consultations

1. Dr. Smith sees a patient in consultation in the hospital at the request of Dr. Jones. He renders an opinion. He then sends a report to Dr. Jones. What code should Dr. Smith use:
    a. Inpatient consultation code √
    b. Initial inpatient hospital care code
    c. Subsequent hospital care code

2. A consultation can be provided:
    a. Only to inpatients
    b. Only to outpatients
    c. To either an inpatient or outpatient √
    d. Only in the emergency room

3. A consultation may be provided by a:
    a. Physician
    b. Other qualified healthcare professional
    c. Non-clinical social worker
    d. Educator
    e. All of these professionals may report consultation codes √

4. Dr. Lewis sees a patient in consultation in the hospital at the request of Dr. Ames. He renders an opinion. He then takes over the management of a portion of the patient's care. What code should Dr. Ames use to bill for his subsequent visits in his office:
    a. Inpatient consultation code
    b. Initial inpatient hospital care code
    c. Subsequent hospital care code
    d. Office/outpatient code (established patient) √
    e. Office/outpatient code (new patient)

5. A mother asks for a consultation to discuss her child. The encounter takes place in the physician's office. This is reported as:
    a. Outpatient consultation
    b. Office or other outpatient service √

6. This patient was seen in the provider's office for a consultation, then admitted by this provider to inpatient/observation care. This is reported using:
    a. Consultation code only
    b. Initial inpatient code only
    c. Both a code for the consultation and a code for initial inpatient care.
    d. Both a code for the consultation and a code for subsequent inpatient care. √

REVIEW – CHAPTER 5
Emergency Services

1. Which one of these emergency services codes does NOT include medical decision making?
   a. 99282
   b. 99283
   c. 99284
   d. 99285
   e. 99288 √

2. Critical care and emergency-level services provided in observation area are reported using:
   a. Only the emergency department code
   b. Only the observation care code √
   c. Both the emergency department code and the observation care code

3. Critical care and emergency department services were provided to a patient on the same date. The emergency services were completed; the patient's condition worsened and critical care services were provided. In this case:
   a. Report only the emergency department code
   b. Report only the critical care code
   c. Report both the emergency department code and the critical care code √

4. For emergency medical systems services (99288), the provider (the individual reporting the code) is located:
   a. In a hospital emergency department or critical care department √
   b. In an ambulance

5. A patient calls her physician about an acute condition. The physician asks her to meet him in the emergency room of a nearby hospital since it is halfway between the patient's home and the physician's office. This is reported using:
   a. An emergency department code
   b. An office/outpatient code √
   c. A consultation code

6. Emergency services were provided to this patient. The patient was then admitted to observation care by the same provider. This is reported using:
   a. An emergency room code only. Add together the time spent in each setting to select the appropriate code.
   b. An observation code only. Add together the time spent in each setting to select the appropriate code. √

227

REVIEW – CHAPTER 6
Neonatal and Pediatric Critical Care Services

1. This patient received critical care services in the Emergency Department. The time providing these services is documented as 2-1/2 hours. The coder should:
   a. List a code from the Emergency Department
   b. List codes 99291 and +99292x3. √
   c. List codes +99292x3 only.
   d. List code 99291x3

2. Which of these critical care codes is NOT selected using minutes spent with patient:
   a. 99291
   b. 99466
   c. 99476 √

3. Which of these critical care codes are reported for non-face-to face services:
   a. 99466
   b. +99467
   c. 99485 √
   d. 99468

4. A critically ill patient, under age 24 months, is being transported from one facility to another, with provider in the vehicle with the patient. These services are reported using:
   a. 99466 √
   b. 99291
   c. +99292
   d. +99486

5. Vascular access procedures are included in:
   a. Pediatric/neonate transport codes
   b. Critical care codes
   c. Inpatient neonatal and pediatric care codes
   d. All of these services √

6. A patient is located in a critical care area but is not currently critically ill. In this case:
   a. Report a critical care code
   b. Report other appropriate code √

7. Codes 99291 and +99292 can be reported for services provided for:
   a. Outpatient care, patient up to 71 months
   b. Critical care transport, patient over 24 months
   c. Inpatient care, patient 6 years or older
   d. These codes can be used In all these circumstances √

8. For reporting face-to-face time for critical care pediatric and newborn transport codes (99466, +99467), begin counting time when:
   a. The physician assumes primary responsibility for a patient at the referring facility √
   b. When the facility accepts responsibility for the patient from the patient
   c. When the physician enters the transport vehicle
   d. When the patient enters the transport vehicle

9. For reporting non-face-to-face time for critical care pediatric and newborn transport codes (99485, +99486), begin counting time when:
   a. When the physician enters the transport vehicle
   b. When the patient enters the transport vehicle
   c. When the provider has first contact with specialized transport team (in the transporting vehicle) √
   d. When the patient's care is handed over to the receiving facility

10. A critically ill pediatric patient is transferred from one facility to another on the same date. The receiving physician at the new facility reports:
    a. Codes 99468, 99471 or 99475 as appropriate √
    b. Codes 99291-99292

11. Two providers are performing critical care services during the same time period. The providers are of different specialties and neither are reporting per day critical care services. In this case:
    a. Only one provider can report critical care codes
    b. Neither provider can report critical care codes
    c. Each provider reports their own critical care codes √

12. Codes 99291, +99292 can be used in any of these settings EXCEPT:
    a. Outpatient settings
    b. Inpatient settings
    c. Patient transport; provider is in vehicle with patient
    d. Patient transport; provider is not in vehicle with patient √

Neonatal and Pediatric Intensive Care Services

1. Some neonatal services overlap with services associated with critical care codes. A service included in both neonatal and critical care codes is:
   a. Heat maintenance
   b. Oral or nasogastric tube placement √
   c. Laboratory and oxygen monitoring
   d. Enteral and/or parenteral nutritional adjustments

2. Sometimes a patient will receive both intensive care and critical care on the same date from providers who are in the same group practice. In this case, report:
   a. Critical care code only √
   b. A critical care code and an intensive care code
   c. Intensive care code only

3. Dr. A provides intensive care. By the next day, the patient no longer needs intensive care, although the baby is still ill. Dr A transfers the infant to Dr. B within the same facility (but not the same group) to provide critical care services. Dr. B reports:
   a. Initial or subsequent critical care √
   b. Subsequent intensive care
   c. Subsequent hospital care
   d. Initial hospital care

4. Most neonatal and pediatric intensive care codes are reported by current body weight. The exception is:
   a. 99477 √
   b. 99478
   c. +99489
   d. 99480

5. A patient may receive intensive care on one day, then be discharged to a lower level of service, but then readmitted to intensive care. For the day of readmission to intensive care, use codes:
   a. Initial intensive care 99477
   b. Subsequent intensive care 99478-99480 √
   c. Initial hospital inpatient services 99231-99333

6. Which of these elements in NOT part of neonatal and pediatric intensive care services:
   a. Patient is critically ill √
   b. Patient requires intensive observation
   c. Patient requires frequent interventions

REVIEW – CHAPTER 8
Nursing Facility Services

1. For E/M coding, a psychiatric residential treatment facility is considered:
   a. An observation care unit
   b. A rest home
   c. Emergency room care
   d. a nursing facility √

2. This patient has been in a nursing facility for 6 months. She is now being released to her home. The coder should select a code for:
   a. Initial service
   b. Subsequent service
   c. Discharge service √
   d. Prolonged service

3. Nursing facility services include a new element in medical decision making. This new element, multiple morbidities requiring intensive management, is used only in this category of MDM:
   a. Number and complexity of problems addressed √
   b. Amount and/or complexity of data to be reviewed
   c. Risk of complication and/or morbidity or mortality of patient management

4. For initial skilled nursing care, the service must be provided by:
   a. Physician √
   b. Clinical staff
   c. Other qualified healthcare professional
   d. Advance care nurse

5. A patient was first seen in the hospital emergency room and then admitted to nursing facility. In this case:
   a. Report both the emergency room and nursing facility codes √
   b. Report only the emergency department code
   c. Report only the nursing facility code

6. A patient was seen for a consultation in the physician's office and then admitted to a nursing facility. In this case:
   a. Report both the outpatient consultation and an initial nursing facility code
   b. Report both the outpatient consultation and a subsequent nursing facility code √
   c. Report only the outpatient consultation code
   d. Report only the initial nursing facility code

7. All of these services are reported with nursing facilities codes EXCEPT:
   a. Care plan oversight √
   b. Skilled nursing facilities
   c. Intermediate care facility for individuals with intellectual disabilities
   d. Psychiatric residential treatment center

Home or Residence Services

1. Home or residence codes are NOT used for services provided in:
    a. Private residence
    b. Group home
    c. Residential substance abuse facility
    d. Intermediate care facility for individuals with intellectual disabilities √

2. A patient is seen in his home for an initial consultation. In this case:
    a. Report an outpatient consultation code √
    b. Report an inpatient consultation code
    c. Report an outpatient consultation code and a home or residence code

3. If selecting a home or residence code using time, count:
    a. Time spent with patient and time spent going to and from the patient's home
    b. Time spent with patient only √
    c. Time is not part of these codes

REVIEW – CHAPTER 10
Prolonged Services

1. Prolonged services codes 99358 and +99359 can only be reported for services provided:
    a. On day of related face-to-face services with patient
    b. On day other than day of related face-to-face services with patient √
    c. On either day of or day before or after the day of a related face-to-face service with patient

2. Prolonged services codes +99415 and +99416 can only be reported for services provided:
    a. In an office or outpatient setting √
    b. In an inpatient or observation setting
    c. In either an office or inpatient/observation setting

3. Prolonged services codes +99418 and +99417 can only be reported for services provided:
    a. Face-to-face only
    b. Non-face-to-face only
    c. Either or both face-to-face and non-face-to-face √

4. Sometimes an E/M service is provided, with prolonged services, and also other services such as a test or diagnostic procedure. In this case:
    a. Include the other services in counting the prolonged services time
    b. Do not include the other services in counting the prolonged services time √

5. A new patient was seen in a face-to-face encounter with clinical staff in the office setting (99205) under the supervision of a physician. The encounter lasted 2 hours. In this case, report code:
    a. 99205, +99415, +99416
    b. 99205, +99415 √
    c. 99205, +99416

6. A provider reviewed test results the day following a face-to-face visit with a patient. The review time was for 80 minutes. In this case:
    a. 99358
    b. 99358 and +99359 √
    c. 99358 and +99359x2

REVIEW – CHAPTER 11
Preventive Medicine Services

1. When a physician performs an E/M preventive care service, the extent of the exam is determined by the:
   a. Patient's age √
   b. Patient's gender
   c. Patient's gender and age
   d. Length of time since patient's last examination

2. Which of the following is **NOT** true about preventive medicine codes:
   a. Documentation must include the patient's age
   b. Documentation must include whether the patient is new or established to this practice
   c. Codes include counseling if done
   d. All of these statements are true √

3. Preventive medicine codes do **NOT** include:
   a. A comprehensive examination
   b. Counseling regarding risk factor reduction
   c. Routine vaccinations √
   d. Ordering of lab tests

4. A preventive medicine service is provided:
   a. When the patient has a documented illness
   b. Only for infants
   c. At the same time as a diagnostic procedure
   d. When the patient is not sick √

5. Counseling and risk factor reduction codes include:
   a. Examination
   b. Time
   c. Counseling only √
   d. Ordering laboratory tests

6. Behavioral change intervention codes are **NOT** reported for:
   a. Smoking cessation counseling
   b. Alcohol abuse intervention counseling
   c. Substance abuse screening
   d. Group counseling for these behaviors √

7. Which of these services include a comprehensive history and examination?
   a. Preventive care services √
   b. Counseling and risk factor reduction
   c. Behavioral change intervention
   d. All of these services include a comprehensive history and examination

Services Provided by Interdisciplinary Teams

1. Care plan oversight services are reported by time:
   a. Per day
   b. Per month √
   c. In minutes

2. Transitional care management codes are selected based on:
   a. Calendar days since face-to-face visit
   b. Level of MDM
   c. Level of MDM and date of first face-to-face visit. √
   d. Location patient is being transferred to
   e. Location patient is being transferred from

3. A patient in an Alzheimer's facility is receiving care plan oversight. The oversight is reported using these codes:
   a. 99374, 99375 √
   b. 99377, 99378
   c. 99379, 99380

4. Transitional care is provided to a patient after discharge. The service includes high complexity MDM and the provider reports code 99496. The first communication with the patient must occur:
   a. Within 7 calendar days of discharge √
   b. Within 8 calendar days of discharge
   c. Within 14 calendar days of discharge

5. Medical team conferences that require presence of a physician is reported using code:
   a. 99366
   b. 99367 √
   c. 99368

6. A medical team conference requires at least:
   a. Minimum of 3 providers from different specialties or disciplines. √
   b. Minimum of 3 providers from same specialty or disciplines.
   c. Only 1 provider
   d. Minimum of 4 providers from same or different specialties or disciplines.

REVIEW – CHAPTER 13

Care Management Services

1. Care management services includes 3 categories. Which of the following do **NOT** include a separate category of codes:
   a. Chronic care management
   b. Complex chronic care management
   c. Principal care management
   d. Care planning √

2. The difference between chronic care management codes and complex chronic care management codes is:
   a. The number of chronic conditions
   b. The time the conditions are expected to last
   c. Requirement for MDM √

3. Principal care management codes 99426-99427 can be reported by:
   a. Physicians only
   b. Qualified health care professional only
   c. Clinical staff under supervision of physicians or qualified health care professional √
   d. Physicians, qualified health care professional or clinical staff

4. A specific level of MDM is required for:
   a. Chronic care management
   b. Complex chronic care management √
   c. Principal care management
   d. Chronic care and complex chronic care management

5. Principal care services code +99427 can be reported:
   a. Once each calendar month
   b. As many times as appropriate during a calendar month
   c. Reported no more than twice per calendar month. √

6. A care plan should be updated/revised:
   a. At least annually. √
   b. Updated every month.
   c. Updated every week.

7. Do **NOT** report chronic care management codes +99437, 99491 with transitional care codes 99495-99496 within:
   a. 45 days
   b. The same calendar month √
   c. The same calendar week
   d. The same 24 hours

REVIEW – CHAPTER 14

Behavioral/Mental Health Services

1. These codes can only be reported every 180 days:
   a. Cognitive assessment and care plan services √
   b. General behavioral health integration care management
   c. Psychiatric collaborative care management

2. General behavioral health integration care management codes can **NOT** be reported during the same month as:
   a. Psychiatric collaborative care management √
   b. Chronic management services
   c. Advance care planning
   d. Counseling, risk factor reduction

3. Psychiatric collaborative care management services include several different types of providers. Which of the following providers administer validated rating scales:
   a. Health care professionals
   b. Behavioral health care managers √
   c. Psychiatric consultants

4. General behavioral health integration care management services are provided by:
   a. Clinical staff √
   b. Physician or other qualified health care professional
   c. Advance practice nurse

5. For psychiatric collaborative care management, the psychiatric consultant communicates directly with:
   a. Treating physician or other QHP
   b. The behavioral health care manager √
   c. The patient

6. The level of medical decision making for cognitive assessment and care plan services is:
   a. Straightforward
   b. Low
   c. Moderate or high √
   d. No MDM is required

7. The cognitive assessment and care management services codes include a long list of included services. These codes can be reported:
   a. If six or more of these services are performed
   b. If any of these services are performed
   c. Only if all of these services are performed. √

Electronic and Telephone Services

1. An E/M service was provided for a patient using an online digital method, in this case email. Five days later, a face-to-face visit for a related condition was provided. In this case:
   a. Add together the time for each service. Report only the online digital E/M service √
   b. Report only the face-to-face visit
   c. Report both the online digital E/M service and the face-to-face visit

2. For telephone services codes, the call must be initiated by:
   a. The provider calling the patient
   b. The provider calling the patient's guardian
   c. The patient or guardian calling the provider √

3. For interprofessional telephone/internet or EHR consultations, the services involve:
   a. The patient and a provider
   b. Two physicians or other qualified health care professional √
   c. Two patients

4. Code 99451 (interprofessional telephone/internet or EHR consultations), the services include:
   a. A consultation with verbal and written report
   b. A consultation with verbal report only
   c. A consultation with written report only √
   d. Consultation and referral services only

5. When calculating time for an online digital service:
   a. Stop counting time 7 days after inquiry √
   b. Start counting time when provider and patient begin online conversation
   c. Stop counting time 14 days following patient's initial contact.
   d. Start counting time 10 days after inquiry.

6. A telephone services code cannot be reported if:
   a. If the patient is seen 48 hours after the call (routine visit).
   b. If an E/M service related to the reason for the call occurs within 2 weeks of the call.
   c. If the patient is seen for the next available urgent visit appointment √
   d. Six weeks following a minor procedure.

REVIEW – CHAPTER 16

1. This code is reported once per episode of care:
   a. Code 99454
   b. Code 99453 √
   c. Code 99091
   d. Code 99474

2. For digitally stored data service/remote physiologic monitoring, the collection and interpretation of data are reported using code:
   a. 99453
   b. 99454
   c. 99091√
   d. 99473

3. For use of the data collected digitally or through remote physiological monitoring for treatment decisions concerning a specific patient, use codes:
   a. 99453-99457
   b. 99457, +99458√
   c. 99473-99474

4. Sometimes the patient collects their own blood pressure data. This is reported using code(s):
   a. 99453, 99454
   b. 99091
   c. 99473, 99474√

5. Teaching a patient to use the device for monitoring is reported using code(s):
   a. 99453, 99473√
   b. 99454, 99474
   c. 99091

6. Code 99457 is reported for services:
   a. Once per episode of care
   b. Once every 30 days
   c. First 20 minutes√
   d. First 30 minutes

REVIEW – CHAPTER 17
Other Services

1. A provider is asked to "stand by" for another provider, and then is called in the provide face-to-face services to that patient. In that case:
    a. Report the stand-by service only
    b. Report the face-to-face service only √
    c. Report codes for both the stand-by and the face-to-face service.

2. Newborn care services are provided to patients 28 days or younger who:
    a. Are normal (no apparent abnormal conditions) √
    b. Require critically ill services
    c. Require intensive care services

3. Disability services code 99450 includes all of these services EXCEPT:
    a. Completion of a medical history following a life insurance form
    b. Collection of blood sample and/or urinalysis
    c. Measurement of height, weight, and blood pressure
    d. Completion of workman's compensation forms √

4. Advance care planning services do **NOT** include:
    a. Health care proxy
    b. Living will
    c. Management of an active problem √
    d. Counseling and completion of appropriate forms

CPT Modifiers and Symbols

1. The physician provided an E/M services during a post-operative period for a condition unrelated to the reason for the surgery. The code should:
    a. Use a modifier 23 on the E/M code
    b. Use a modifier 24 on the E/M code √
    c. Use a modifier 25 on the E/M code
    d. Not use any modifier

2. The physician provided an unrelated E/M service on the same day as a surgery. In this case, the coder should:
    a. Use a modifier 24 on the E/M code
    b. Use a modifier 25 on the E/M code √
    c. Use a modifier 24 on the surgical code
    d. Use a modifier 25 on the surgical code

3. Dr. White removed John's gallbladder. John is a Medicare patient. This procedure has a 90 day global package. He comes into the office 10 days after the surgery to see Dr. White because of a problem in his knee (an E/M service). The modifier used in this case is:
    a. 24 √
    b. 25
    c. 26
    d. 27

4. The physician provided an unrelated E/M service on the same day as a surgery.
    a. Use a modifier 57 on the E/M code
    b. Use a modifier 24 on the E/M code
    c. Use a modifier 25 on the E/M code √
    d. Not use any modifier

5. The symbol ▲ means:
    a. This guideline has been revised this year.
    b. This code is out of numerical order.
    c. This code is new this year.
    d. This code was revised this year √

6. The patient was brought in by her mother to the physician's office. The child was complaining of ear pain. The provider did an E/M service and determine the patient had an ear infection. The provider scheduled an insertion of a ventilating tube next week (code 69436). The provider reports:
    a. An E/M code with a modifier 57 and code 69436.
    b. An E/M code without a modifier and code 69436. √
    c. An E/M code only.
    d. Code 69436 only.

Definitions of CPT Terms

1. Dr. A is on-call for Dr. B. Dr. A sees an established patient of Dr. B. Dr. A has never seen this patient before. Dr. A reports the visit as:
   a. Subsequent service
   b. New patient
   c. Initial service
   d. Established patient √

2. A new patient is defined as a patient who has not seen the physician or any physician of the same specialty in the same group practice:
   a. Within the last year
   b. Within the last 2 years
   c. Within the last 3 years √
   d. Within the last 4 years

3. A patient has been seeing Dr. A, a dermatologist in a multispecialty practice, for years. The patient then sees Dr. B, an orthopedist, who belongs to the same practice. His last visit with Dr. A was one year ago. For the visit with Dr. B, the patient is considered a:
   a. New patient √
   b. Established patient
   c. Initial patient
   d. Subsequent patient

4. Physician A asks Physician B to take over care for a specific problem for this patient. This is referred to as a:
   a. Transitional care management
   b. Transfer of care √
   c. Shared visit
   d. Concurrent service

5. A qualified healthcare professional (QHP) may be:
   a. Certified nurse midwife
   b. Nurse practitioner
   c. Physician assistant
   d. Physician
   e. All of the above √

6. Codes that are reported per day can be selected:
   a. Using time only
   b. Using MDM only
   c. Using cumulative time or MDM elements for the whole date √

INDEX

Other Books by This Author

ICD-10-CM Coding Guidelines Made Easy

ICD-10-PCS Coding Guidelines Made Easy

Changes to ICD-10-CM and ICD-10-PCS Code Books
2024

Look for annual updates each fall (or as needed)!

Visit me on Facebook – Tropin's Medical Coding,
https://www.facebook.com/codingteacher

Visit my YouTube Channel for coding videos on ICD-10-CM,
ICD-10-PCS and CPT® codes –
Tropin's Medical Coding Made Easy
https://www.youtube.com/channel/UCIZMO2J4goul_BBQg5lBMnw

Made in the USA
Columbia, SC
16 May 2024

35734153R00135